# THE HISTORY OF VACCINES

THE UNTOLD REALITIES AND THE THEORIES THAT SUPPORT THEM

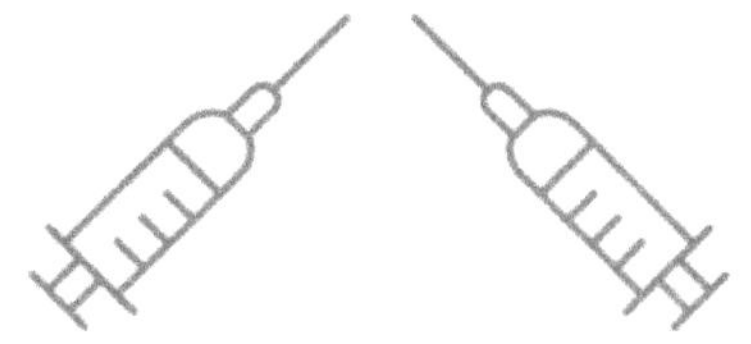

By

Rachel Banura

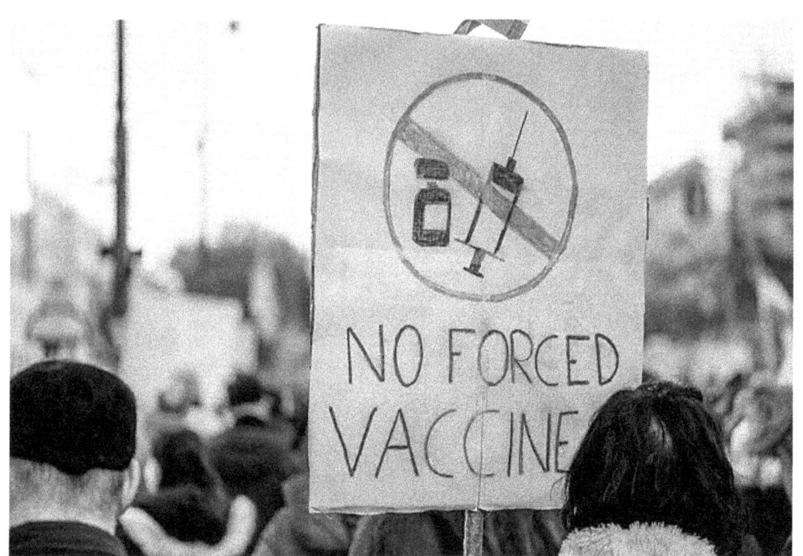

November 20, 2021



ISBN: 979-8-9991838-1-1

"Come in, madam! Be not afraid! Does this little one belong to you? So, so! What a lovely babe! Truly a young hero! A perfect ideal of health!" exclaims the vaccine-physician to the trembling mother who is full of doubts and misgivings. "Here! Read yourself; read the new law, provided by the modern legislators of Athens. It says: Vaccination does not do the least harm!" This overpowers the last gleam of God-given instinct in the doubting mother-soul; the snow-white, pure little arms are bared and offered, and the poison 6—12—18—24 times incised; for it is of acknowledged importance, "that the vaccine-poison be forced into the unwilling body in SUFFICIENT quantity! THE MORE THE BETTER!!"

Dr. C.G.G. Nittinger's Evils of Vaccination 1856

"Every Physician of experience has met with numerous cases of cutaneous eruptions, erysipelas, and syphilis, which were directly traceable to vaccination, and if these could all be collected and presented in one report, they would form a more terrible picture than the worst than has ever been drawn to portray the horrors of small-pox."

Vaccination by Robert A. Gunn 1882

"Now, let us reckon with vaccination. What service has it rendered humanity? It has shackled the organic functions, it has suppressed the vital force, it has infinitely multiplied the most terrible maladies, pulmonary consumption, scrofula, cancer, insanity, rickets, paralysis. It has even given birth to croup, and, more particularly, to internal variola, called typhus fever, which is now more common than eruptive small-pox. Thus, out of a vigorous and powerful nature, it has made the miserable race you see. In a word, it has deranged the mental faculties, corroded the lungs, ulcerated the intestines; it has done all that, and yet—it has not preserved us from Small-Pox."

Dr. Verde-Delisle 1856*

*(the yr. 1856 or possibly a bit later.) The exact publishing date of this work was unknown as only fragments were preserved.

# About this book

This book is designed a bit like an oversized research paper in that there are multiple sights and sources referenced.

At the beginning, and throughout are histories of the start (before the 1800's) of vaccination up to the present.

Also included are stories from families who have experienced side-effects and damage of all kinds from vaccines which are included very close, if not exactly as they have been shared publicly.

There are several charts included along with data from various websites including news articles, interviews, videos and even written transcripts of speeches no longer available on the original platforms.

There are, in the Appendix section, a great number of resources including websites, links to videos, Facebook profiles, books and articles for further research and information and suggestions for understanding your rights and creating exemption requests.

This is designed as an informational and research tool to get you started on your journey of discovering the truth about the history of vaccines and created to share the many voices who have a story to tell about the reality of vaccination that is quite different than the widely accepted and broadly acknowledged narrative.

This is NOT my personal story, only. It is a broad and unified consensus about vaccination from a wide variety of sources that I believe desperately needs to be shared. It does also contain my personal thoughts and opinions on the matter.

Disclaimer: I do not claim to be a medical professional. I do not claim to be an authority on vaccines or medical procedures. This book is for Informational Purposes only. My aim is to share already established history, data and information, voices both professional and personal in a concise and cohesive manner.

# Acknowledgements & Special Thanks

The creation of this book is predicated on the time and efforts of countless authors, doctors, scientists and others who have ensured the preservation of texts and histories that would otherwise have been lost to the public.

Much of the heart and soul of this book's content come from the shared stories from the lives of the parents and families of the vaccine injured children and their courage and desire to see truth revealed and others spared the horrors and loss they endured.

Thanks to Children's Health Defense, Circle of Mammas, Sarah Peterson, and a great many others referenced in the Appendix section and elsewhere throughout the book for the creation, accumulation and sharing of websites, studies, news articles, charts and data as well as ingredients and other information on vaccines that are referenced throughout this book.

It must also be acknowledged that those who continued to share their stories, and others' stories were the fire that inspired this book in the first place and its continuation, despite time constraints and difficulties.

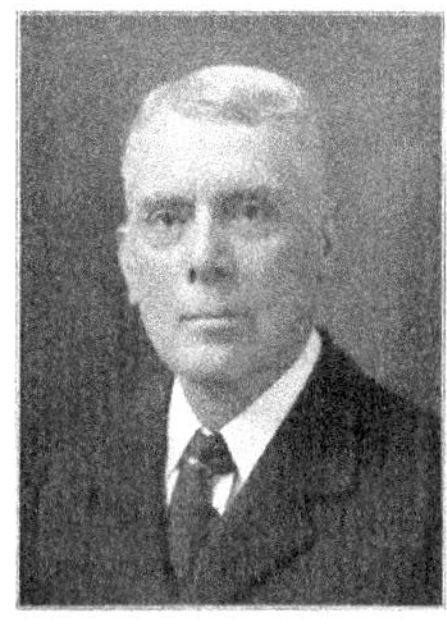

Thanks to Physicians, present and past, like Charles Creighton, whose books and works on the History of Vaccination began the process which inspired me to write this book many years ago.

Thank you, most of all, to all who advocate for those who were impacted by vaccines and your continued and tireless efforts to bring awareness to this most vital area of health.

# Dedication

This book is dedicated to the lives of those whose suffering and courage paved the way for truth and the creation of an alternative narrative than one which has no problem exploiting others for the sake of personal gain and power.

It is also dedicated to my children whose presence makes me overflow with gratefulness to be a mom and causes my heart to ache for other moms who loved their children no less, yet lost them, or a part of them, due to the poison in vaccines.

# Table of Contents

# An Almost Entirely Forgotten History

## Introduction

One of the worst things that can happen to our current generation is the loss of previous histories. Truly, of all the things that set us apart from ignorant or even animal-like beings, knowing where we came from and who we are is at the top of the list. Also, knowing where we went wrong, learning from our past experiences and not repeating them are also high on that list. This book is driven by two things: a desire to inform and prevent more damage from occurring and a desire to document things that should not be forgotten, hidden or overlooked.

I have been studying the history of health for decades (and the history of vaccines for years), trying to research, observe, put to the test, and prove what I believe is true in the world of health. While I do have many theories about health, most of what I'll be sharing in this book is not my own ideas but others' stories and documents from our past that have already confirmed facts that most people currently Do Not Know. Why? Because the truth about vaccines is Not part of the current, medically accepted narrative, and because finding the truth is something you really do have to search for, and, as I have discovered from diving into the topic, much of the information is well hidden, or simply not there.

As a mom, my greatest driving force for pressing on with this book, despite time constraints and being a full-time mom, are the stories of the little lives lost or forever maimed from the poison in vaccines. My heart is aching for other moms, children, babies, families and people who are just trying to live their lives and do the best they can but are being fed lies in an area that could literally kill them or just slowly, and utterly unnecessarily, weaken their immune system.

We are truly living in unprecedented times, particularly in the amount of information available at the push of a button, or more accurately, the swipe of a screen. Simultaneously, the proliferation of misinformation being promulgated across the country through various media channels is staggering. Particularly, as we will be discussing in this book, in Health Care, and more specifically, in Vaccination. The narrative surrounding vaccination is perplexing, frustrating, and grievous for me, because what has become widely known (about vaccines) and commonly practiced is dead wrong, and widely hurtful. I think more and more people are beginning to realize this, and hopefully many more will continue to do so.

If you still believe that every story being told by the popular media today is true, then you will likely not have ears for anything I have to say in this book. But, if you are reading this, you are probably already on a path with the desire to discover the Truth. Even if that Truth is unpopular or difficult to find. I truly hope this book can be a tool to equip the readers with enough information to convince anyone with an open mind of both the evil and futility of vaccination.

In the first part of this book, I want to begin with some of the earliest histories of vaccination and relay them in a concise and understandable manner. While I draw from many different resources both on the history and science of vaccination up through the present, I want to include Data, Stories, Facts (about vaccines, ingredients and reactions etc.) along with some discussion on the theories and ideas that I believe need to be re-evaluated and questioned.

Finding books on the earliest history of vaccination and attaining them was a challenge, along with the many sites, articles and stories that are well-hidden by the most popular web searches and acclaimed information hubs. I wanted to start at the beginning to show how the narrative began, and how it has similarly continued. I will share many of the sources I gathered and used as well as a few I haven't but believe also have valuable information, in the Appendix Section. I really do hope it can be a tool that will help bring freedom and awareness in this area. I am so happy you are reading this and hope that this information can avert a great and unnecessary evil for you and your loved ones!

I do believe that if information, such as is contained in the pages of this book could simply be known to the public, the hold the Vaccine and Pharmaceutical industry has on the lives of those it exploits for profit would be obliterated. For who could not be angered by a forceful injection of toxins into the whole body of an innocent child and watch them forever be wounded, maimed, brain infected or even killed because their vulnerable system was directly impacted by toxins being pushed through their skin and into their bloodstream to permanently alter their immune system, bodily organs, brain, nervous and/or other systems with **substances designed to be dangerous or toxic**. Designed to be so injurious to your system that it never can forget the trauma enforced upon it. Indeed, and usually by a loving parent and well-meaning physician who are being fed a lie (and others simply a paycheck) all because of a THEORY that became accepted into our culture over two hundred years ago by the authority (not science) of so-called "experts" whose primary concerns were not the well-being of their fellow man. Despite the data and records and cries that should have proved the failure of vaccination centuries ago, we will find many of the same explanations, reasoning, excuses and pretense that existed then, plaguing our institutions to this day.

When a previously healthy child complains of pain in the head or abdomen, continues their screams for days, behaves lethargically, stops responding or taking an interest in what they did just a day ago, loses their appetite or desire to play, stares mindlessly into space, can no longer handle the stress of school or daily activities... the list goes on and on... still, we are told that it is not because vaccines are harmful and deadly or that the poor child's immune system is overwhelmed. Instead, we are told that it is "all coincidence." Yet, denying (and often hiding) the obvious (or what should be) for the sake of an already established belief has been a large part of the continuing saga that has been the practice of vaccination.

The Truth, the large corporations (the ones funding so much of the medical institutions) are hiding at all costs and desperately do not want you to know is that ALL this is **completely unnecessary**! That vaccines never had anything helpful to offer and they still do not. That the decline in deaths from disease had nothing to do with vaccines. This is the TRUTH that should be obvious, but that no one in either the medical world or political arena is willing to say.

The devastation of the COVID-19 vaccination had, as its blessing, the dangers and problems of vaccination made so obvious that many who were faithful vaccinators began to see its evils. The whole purpose of this book is to prove to you, beyond any reasonable doubt, that ALL Vaccinations, indeed both the theories that support their existence and the claims of their efficacy and safety, were, from their very inception, a LIE. History has already proven that vaccination (or inoculation as it first was called) is an utterly useless (and hurtful) practice that never did, at any point in time, protect the receiver against future disease or strengthen one's immune system in any way. If vaccines do neither of these, then what is their advantage?

Now, this is a broad topic that has spanned many diseases over many eras, and not all vaccinations are the same, yet all have proved injurious, to some degree or another. There is no book that could contain EVERYTHING there is to know or understand on this subject, and this book is far from comprehensive, but my goal is to provide pieces and summaries from many different sources: documents, stories, data, information and voices on the subject that ought to be more than enough to provide a sufficient framework on the subject, along with the resources to dig deeper and go further than this book. I hope you will at least allow me to present a fuller picture of the OTHER SIDE of the story, for it has, up till now, been presented very one-sided in the majority of universally accepted "authorities on the matter."

I will state that I am in no way claiming to be a medical professional or authority on vaccines. Everything I share will be for Informational Purposes Only, and I invite (and implore) you to not take my word for anything written or shared in this book. I believe an honest approach to searching out the reality of vaccination will prove itself. I hope that you will question and search out all the claims made in this book. The desire is to record, share and declare TRUTH that has been pushed aside and overlooked for far too long.

In the first part of this book, I want to share some of the earliest histories that I have compiled. We will begin with where it all started.

# CHAPTER 1

## THE RISE OF THE JENNERIAN DOCTRINE

(Charles Creighton on Jenner and Vaccination)

A significant part of my research was the discovery of a renowned Physician during the inception of vaccination and one of its most vocal critics and observers. While reading a book about the Influenza virus, I saw that it mentioned a Dr. Charles Creighton (and not in a favorable light). If you have ever researched the topic, you will find the overwhelming majority (if not all) of the resources on both the Germ Theory of Disease and Vaccination are very one-sided. The theory is proclaimed as fact by everyone in agreement with, or who promotes what you could call, "The Mainstream Medical Narrative" which stems from what we talk about later in this book called, "The Germ Theory of Disease." Yet, to many, not so heralded, yet brilliant and wise physicians, the ludicrous nature and realities surrounding the practice of inoculation, and its supporting theories, was so much more obvious than its so called "success." Charles Creighton was one such physician, and he wrote extensively on his observations of the development of inoculation/vaccination in the days of its creation throughout its development and growing use and popularity.

Most of this chapter comes from Dr. Creighton's observations and recordings and is the most thorough writings I have found of its history (though we will discuss others as well). For the sake of time and conciseness, I will be sharing a small summary and few stories, but for those of you who would like a more thorough reading, stories and history, I invite you to read Dr. Charles Creighton's book: *Jenner and Vaccination, a Strange Chapter of Medical History* (this is the only book of His on the subject of Vaccines that I have been able to access, though not the only one he has written). *The Evils of Vaccination, with a Protest Against Its Legal Enforcement* by George S. Gibbs is a short, but very valuable manuscript, and Dr. C.G.G. Nittinger's *Evils of Vaccination* is also a great treatise on the subject. Also, *Vaccination* (It's Fallacies and Evils) by Robert A. Gunn.

I apologize for any difficulty with understanding the following chapter, as the words and language are two hundred years old, but I wanted to include actual quotes and data from the original work to share here.

One of my goals with this book and this chapter is to deliver a proper history of the development of vaccines along with the opinions and writings of those whose voices on the matter should never have been forgotten or discarded. Dr. Creighton was both a renowned physician and a brilliant scholar, yet you won't find his name in any modern textbook or likely have heard of his 22 extensive and comprehensive works in health and medicine. Of his character, I think it worth saying, that I find in Dr. Creighton that same industrious, logical and scientific mind that you find in true professionals, that exemplify the passion and hard work that only come from love of their work and the pursuit of truth and discovery. Edward Jenner, on the other hand, exemplifies that same sort of spirit that I have found (in studying different histories) common in those who often lack the "genius" and yet somehow succeed in taking the limelight. Jenner went from delivering his essays on his observations of studying the cuckoo bird, the greater parts of which were best remembered as "a tissue of inconsistencies and absurdities"(Creighton p.17). Yet this launched him into the Royal Academy. Here he went on to promote his idea about a milkmaid with cowpox sores and the proposition that people who suffered this disease seemed to be forever exempt from smallpox, with no well-documented or scientifically sound argument.

As time went on, Creighton notes, "the medical leaders in London had come to form a tolerably accurate personal estimate of Jenner and might have come, in course of time to form an equally accurate estimate of his cowpox doctrine. It was an open secret in the profession that the great discoverer was a disappointing person at close quarters. He was vain, perpetuate, crafty and greedy. He had more of grandiloquence and bounce than of solid attainments (p. 338)."

So, it seems to be the repeatable essence of history, that the character of the one who offers such a hurtful theory to the world (rather like the indomitable disposition of Carl Marx) becomes in hindsight a great mystery that the world so overwhelmingly and to its great demise, listens to such advice.

## The Rise of "Smallpox of the Cow"

Jenner gathered his idea of cow pox as a protective from a few tales he had collected and submitted them to the Royal Society (of science) along with a drawing of a girl with sores on her hands and arms. Jenner named this cowpox *Variolae Vaccinae* which in Latin means: Smallpox of the Cow (a deception in nomenclature for sure). Over and over Dr. Creighton points out that there never was such a thing, truly, as smallpox of the cow, and smallpox had nothing in common with the malady of cows but the "verbal jingle" containing the term "pox"(p. 23). It was amazing, or perhaps shocking, to see people so readily accept the idea. Although there always remained those medical doctors and farmers who knew the true nature of each [smallpox and the inflamed udders of cows] and the laughable concept of not just the name but many other of Jenner's propositions. Notably, the Royal Society rejected his first submission. Yet Jenner went about to revise his paper and begin collecting "proof" for his theory. So, on May 14th Jenner took the initial steps into proving his theory by taking some fluid from a large vesicle from the arm of a milk maid, Sarah Nelmes, and inoculating it into the arm of 8-year-old James Phipps. Later, on July 2nd he inoculated him with smallpox (p. 36).

It is certainly worth noting that the boy, James Phipps, who became his poster child was observed by Creighton, and indeed Jenner himself, to be scrofulous (a diseased condition of the lymphatic system) and likely had Tuberculosis. “Poor Phipps,” as Jenner called him, was inoculated some 20 times and never “took”(p.46 & 126) meaning that he had no visible reaction. Creighton relays that his “lymph system was already full and immobile” and was past the ability to produce any more sores.

This is a common occurrence (rarely talked about now): that once the body's cellular (as the Lymph System) and more superficial boundaries (like the skin) have been breached enough, disease becomes rampant in the inner organs such as in Tuberculosis. If he was suffering already from T.B. it was likely he was past the season for a skin breakout detox reaction. Tuberculosis was one of those diseases that we later see on the rise as inoculation becomes rampant. It is a disease often seen in those who have already been afflicted with smallpox, measles, or a similar outbreak of diseases, but more often in those who have been vaccinated with toxins, especially when vaccinated multiple times.

The fact that one boy did not react to a smallpox inoculation is hardly ample proof that the previous inoculation succeeded in providing protection from disease. Especially when a great many other failures surrounded this “success,” as we’ll soon see.

A noteworthy declaration of Dr. Creighton (p. 155), "The apologetics of vaccination began in the mind of Jenner before his project was given to the world. The years of patient observing and proving which have been the subject of so much rhetorical nonsense on the part of so many otherwise sane persons were really a few years of indolent casting about by Jenner with the means of meeting the obvious objections to the scientific whitewashing and professional adoption which he intended for the vulgar cowpox legend. All Jenner's medical neighbors knew that there was nothing more in the legend than the verbal Jingle of cowpox /smallpox just as dog-rose and hound's-tongue are charms against mad dogs or remedies for their bites. The alleged immunity of poxed milkers from smallpox they knew to be a mere popular delusion, which did not find the smallest justification in the experience of any medical man who had seen much practice among the class of milkers. That was the commonsense obstacle to Jenner's fanciful ambition to see cowpox inoculation substituted for the ordinary inoculation of the time period. Jenner resolved to circumvent that obstacle, and all other obstacles of the evidential sort, by calmly asserting that the ordinary spontaneous cowpox was spurious, and that the sort of cowpox which alone gave immunity from smallpox was a derivative of horse grease." (More on this later)

## The Tests

Besides the famous non-reaction of James Phipps, *The Inquiry* contained two or at the most three other children who had variolous tests performed, by his assistant, as Jenner rushed to have his report printed. Upon his return, he applied the test to one other [previously vaccinated] child who produced an eruption and fever (p. 127).

Though Jenner did not inoculate [with smallpox] any cases in Stroud, the doctors there tested all 10 cases [of those who had been previously vaccinated] and found that only one adult, "whose vaccination had not held", stood the variolous test, while the other 9 took smallpox in some form.

Here is a record of one of the physicians, not long after this time, that was boasting his great success, having vaccinated over 200 subjects and declaring up to half of them "protected." Yet what do we find of the actual data reported by his own records??

To sight just a few of several, similar data records.

Case 1, 7-year-old girl successfully vaccinated. Later has smallpox. (fail)
Case 2, her 9 yr. old brother catches smallpox from her. [this alone should dispel the germ protection theory]
Case 3, 5 mo. old Vaccine did not hold. Variolation did.
In cases 4-7 the Variolation failed.
Case 8 & 9, [claims] the vaccine successful. The first one had all

the symptoms including eruptions and fever etc. but by the 22nd day he has no reaction to variolation. The second one breaks out, again, all over on the 29th day with pustules.
Case 10-11, aged 14 wks. and 9 mo. Both were inoculated from the first girl (who had had smallpox), they had all the awful (typical) eruptions and symptoms until day 12. 2 days later they were both variolated with no result.
Case 12-14, results unknown. (p.130-131)

What do you think of such records? I love Creighton's own words on the matter. "What are we to think of the temper of the profession at this time, when a respectable practitioner congratulates the world upon a great discovery with failure staring him in the face from the record of his own experience?" (p.131)

How can one not see the inconsistencies (at the very least)? One is inoculated with Cowpox, then gets smallpox. [FAILURE] Two others are vaccinated [from her]. Half of the variolations [as stated] did not "hold." Some were tested on the 22nd day, others on the 2nd ?? Why do they not consider that at least in some of these, their body was literally just finished with breaking out? [well, that time frame seemed to scream failure let's try a different time frame... how about until we find a moment we can get them inoculated without creating an eruption??]

Another example of some results of a case forwarded to Jenner, from a Dr. Drake on May 9th, 1799, who used cow pox material from Jenner, himself.

"In three of them: a lad aged 17 and two of the Colborne children: one 4 years the other 15 months, the cowpox vesicles came to early maturity and were scabbed under the usual time. The lad was inoculated with smallpox on the 20th December, being the 8th day from his vaccination and the two children on the 21st being, again, the 8th day, they all developed smallpox, both the local pustule and the general eruption with fever. The remaining 2 cases: a lad aged 15 and the third Colborne child aged 2 years and 1/2 were also very related on the 21st December or the 8th day of their vaccination, but these two developed the local pustules only. The reason why they did not have the consecutive fever and general eruption of smallpox will perhaps appear from the peculiar history of their cowpox sores. In the lad W. King, the areola appeared on the 10th day and continued spreading until the 15$^{th}$. On the 18th day the scab which now occupied the center of the vesicle put on the appearance of an eschar with much induration of the tissues, around on the 29th day the eschar separated and left a sore 1/4 of an inch deep which under treatment with mercurial ointment filled up and skinned over in due course. He had meanwhile been tried a second time with smallpox on the 1st of January but resisted it entirely, his cowpox sore being on that day and for a week longer in its eschar stage and his lymphatics doubtless clogged. The case of the child E. Colborne was somewhat similar on the 10th day, her cow pox vesicle was the size of a six-penny piece, mostly a scab with a narrow ring around the margin containing matter. On the 15th day the crust was the margin containing matter. On the 15th day the crust was thrown off and left a small superficial eschar which increased in depth in the next few days. Much inflammation followed in the skin around and two small supervisions broke out a little above the original vaccine puncture each of which reached the size of a shilling. One of them communicating with the original sore. On the 4th of February, being the 52nd day from vaccination, the sores were all healed, and the induration gone. Meanwhile this child had also been tried a second time with smallpox on the 1st of January entirely without effect." (p. 95-96)

A summary of this experiment had reached Jenner, and I quote, "two of them had alarming ulcerations on their arms and these two, whose arms were so dreadfully affected, did not take the smallpox while the other three received it." (So, while these children were literally oozing from one end, they apparently failed to "erupt" at the other end) and for the other three, it was just an all-out failure.

Jenner claimed that the information came to him "too late" to include in his pamphlet.

Before that, a Dr. Thornton, on Dec. 1st, 1798, took matter from the hands of a milkmaid with ulcerations on them (the same way that Jenner had begun, originally) and used it to inoculate Mr. Stanton and his 4 children: from 10 yrs to 10 months in age. It records as follows, (p. 93-94)

"On the third day, the arms of the four children were affected with a kind of "erysipelatous efflorescence" above the point of insertion. About a fortnight after, the punctures began to be covered with a thick crust, from which some ichor was discharged for several days. The inflammation subsided and the scabs fell off about the 20th day. "From the long continued local excitement," Mr. Thornton began to hope that the virus might imperceptively have crept into the habit and proved a security against the variolus infection: but it was not, for when they were tried to see whether the cow pox had made them insusceptible, all the children "received the infection and passed through the stages in the usual slight manner"; the father, whose vaccination had failed altogether was the only one of the five who resisted the smallpox.

"This damning experience of cowpoxing from a source used by Jenner himself and authenticated with full particulars, ought to have raised a suspicion that there was something wrong (p. 94)."

Many of these summaries were published in the *Inquiry* or in the *Medical and Physical Journal*, but Jenner had a way of side-stepping what should have been obvious failures.

As Creighton points out, (p. 97) "at the end of 1798, or six months after the inquiry was published, the case for cowpoxing as a substitute for inoculation with smallpox stood as follows: nearly all the children's arms had ulcerated, some of them to an alarming extent, just as the milker's hands nearly always ulcerated. Jenner neglected the variolous test in some of his cases and got a rather equivocal test in others. The variolous test, when applied by Drake and Hughes in one set of cases, and by Thornton in another, gave a result which was as far as possible from bearing out Jenner's confident assurances. In some medical circles these adverse effects were as well known then as they are now to us in the retrospect; and it is the strongest possible evidence of the good-will, nay, the welcome, extended to Jenner and his innovation, that the fatal objections were not pressed."

I find it fascinating that Creighton states how obvious and well-known the failure (and more specifically the adverse effects) of cowpoxing was in retrospect of a time so far in our past and yet somehow still unknown to us today.

What was now, in 1799, termed Jennerian Vaccination, was taken up by an anatomist and surgeon named Von Sommerring, in conjunction with a Dr. Lehr. The precision with which he records his methods, Creighton calls one of the "best recorded variolous tests in the whole of literature of Vaccination" (p. 226). I include the details here:

"Fourteen vaccinated children were brought together in one place, and all inoculated on the same day with smallpox before witnesses. The smallpox matter was taken fresh from a child's pustules at the third day of their suppurative stage and was inserted by lancet-puncture. The children were kept under observation and inspected from time to time by impartial witnesses. By the second or third day inflammation had arisen at the punctures in them all, and a popular elevation could be felt; on the fourth day all the papules had a zone of redness about half an inch around, and a little yellow fluid at their summits; on the fifth and sixth days, eleven of the fourteen cases showed the papules become pustules, larger or smaller, filled with yellow matter, the remaining three cases having aborted from the popular stage; on the seventh day the redness begun to decline and the pustules to wither; and on the eighth day the redness had disappeared, and the pustules become covered with yellowish-brown semi-transparent crusts. No eruption followed."

Creighton took the account from the Salzburg Journal, and even though all this care was taken to record the process, it omitted to say how soon after vaccination the test was applied. It was the practice during that time, though, to apply the test very soon after: usually the 8-10th day. The absence of an eruption at that point then was no great marvel.

## The New Vaccination

Not long after this, an attempt was made to try to refine the material used for inoculating the patient, to render less of an ulceration. A man named Woodville (p. 101) experimented with lymph taken from the hands of milkmaids and the teats of cows, and much trial and error on hundreds of patients. In some cases, the lymph was passed through several cows, and an attempt was made to use lymph from a vesicle in the very earliest stages of ulcerating. Some success was granted to Woodville during the hundreds of attempts. It seemed he had a way of inoculating his patients in just the right way, or at just the right intervals to receive less ulceration in the arm being inoculated than typical inoculators. Yet, as Dr. Creighton points out, even his great "success stories" are riveted with incorrect data and large amounts of failures that were simply disregarded.

Jenner himself attempted to create a vaccine lymph that produced less violent ulcerations. There was an attempt to create a different sort of lymph from a cow ranging over the "fertile meadows and the veil of Gloucester" versus the typical or what they called, "artificial pampering of cows" that had been previously used. However, even after prolific amounts of diseased cow udders and hundreds more attempts to create some difference of eruption it never proved significant. "See the circular figure," he would explain or the "smooth surface" or the "less pointed shape or peculiar scab" etc. Yet, these noted "differences" from a particular type of vaccination was simply a battle of terms with no real obvious difference in the ulcers or scabs produced. Doctor Woodville was said to be more "acute" in his findings, which, was simply being more honest than Jenner was about the differences in appearance of the scabs which developed from the ulcerations on the arms of those inoculated and those from the teats of cows. (p. 113)

In France, a man named Gatti, began an inoculation technique which, he claimed, offered protection from smallpox without the typical ulcerations, lesions, and fevers etc. that past inoculators had produced. This "new way" of vaccinating was also used in London, England and America. An eminent surgeon named William Bromfield and a Doctor Langton of Salisbury, were some of the few men who opposed the "new way of inoculating." Bromfield was told that "many lost their lives [from smallpox] in Paris, after epidemical frenzy for inoculating in the new way there (which was a fact), which, in general, neither occasioned fever or eruptions." Their fears, though, were less of the evils of vaccination itself and more of the dangers of straying from the previously accepted practice. Well, it might have been a better option if it produced fewer pustules and just as good protection... the only problem was that neither the old nor the "new" way provided protection from smallpox. (p. 137-141)

## The Substitute of Horse Grease

After this, Jenner began using a pox material from horse grease. I quote Doctor Creighton who says, "the advocates of horse grease in 1800 to 1803 as we shall see were under the same illusion from their want of pathological knowledge. The tumid whitish vesicle or bleb on a farrier's or stableman's hand was just the same as that upon a milker's although the cow's pap-pox was far from resembling the horse's greased hocks either in causation, or in development or in issue. The point in common between them was inveterate soreness through filth and neglect; and the infective discharges of each... creating, in due course, a painful and corroding ulcer." (p. 123)

He goes on to say, "it seems well-nigh incredible that medical men with some pretensions to a discriminating knowledge of the processes of disease should have allowed Jenner's bold invention of a "smallpox of the cow" derived from horse-grease to pass into current professional teaching."

## Attenuation

The idea that the matter used and still referred to as cow pox matter (or variolea vacinae) was taken from a host other than a cow should have seemed ludicrous. It should greatly concern us that the common practice (in recent vaccine creations) that attempt to "attenuate a virus", namely: take diseased matter and try to infect other animals (like mice, rats or bats or monkeys or pigs etc.) in an attempt to make the virus itself less "virulent" or milder began with this insanity. Yet all "attenuation" ever truly accomplished was picking up more foreign matter and debris (viral particles) from all these other hosts which ended up bringing more foreign particles (and disease processes) to the body than the original "virus" ever would have to begin with. (We will discuss more about such ideas in the VIRUS chapter.)

## Acceptance

Germany, whose epidemic pushed through a greater inclination to submit their children to the "new inoculation" was one of the first countries to declare that the "period of scrutiny" was over. Enough journals were published, and enough physicians were declaring the "success" and necessity of it. Some professors, like Hecker the Elder at Erfert in 1799, proclaimed that "the old smallpox inoculation, did not make so much progress in the 80 years since its introduction as the Jennerian inoculation with "smallpox of the Cow" has done in two or three years (p. 229)."

Many places, like Bavaria (p.230), received the Jennerian vaccination without qualms or scrutiny, which seemed to be simply on faith alone. Some others, like Vienna (p. 232), made a practical trial beforehand. They pointed out a few things, such as the establishment of "Cow's smallpox" as a new disease, when it was only made so by the invention, by Jenner, of the term, Variolae Vaccinae, and not by any scientific proof. Also, they pointed out that three, and only three, of Jenner's vaccinations had been tested with smallpox, and three was too small a number.

## Excuses

Jenner was a master of finding excuses for why vaccination went wrong (as it often did) and had a great many excuses to draw from: The timing was off, the inoculation matter was not true vaccine lymph, or his favorite word for when vaccination obviously failed (especially if he had administered it himself) was, it was "spurious." Spurious, which Jenner defined this way: "under certain circumstances, the vaccine does not follow its "regular course" in certain subjects and may give rise to a false vaccine which provides no protection from smallpox."

Well, with a definition like that you could call any failure "spurious" and somehow get away with calling the "normal course for vaccination" a success. There was also the "general" vs "local" pustule. A local pustule, or eruption, was expected to occur when a subject was inoculated, but only if what Jenner and others called a "general" pustule showed up could you consider it a true reaction and therefore, if there was no "general pustule" the person could still be considered "protected." Without any real scientific proof or consistencies and utter disregard for any true scientific method, all the conjecture as to what was truly going on in the body was theoretical and built on invented hypotheses.

The conclusion of the previously stated test by Von Sommerring and Dr. Lehi, of the 14 vaccinated children was that "in none of them did the slightest trace of smallpox infection declare itself (p. 235)." This declaration would not have been possible if the criteria were that they had no reaction or pustule at all. For the presence of "local pustules" as they were declared by Jenner and his followers meant nothing, only the presence of the "general eruption."

Another excuse emerged for the failure of a vaccine to "take." As stated in a recent essay on the matter, "The presence of any common eruption, even itch, was well known to prevent the cowpox from taking." Also, from an essay by Burges on the Preparation and Management necessary to Inoculation we read that "cutaneous eruptions render a child an improper subject for inoculation, until those disorders are removed."

Fever was taken as a proof that variolation "took" yet, in another instance (when it raises its inconvenient head) is disregarded as nothing (no indicator of a smallpox disease response). But no excuse was given as often as Jenner's declaration that the vaccine was "Spurious." (P. 243, 244, 248 etc.)

One story stands out in the book about a Dr. Defresne (p. 261), resolving to give the new protective inoculation a try. He received the vaccine on "a thread from Dr, Coindet, one of the Geneva vaccinators, with which he raised a successful vesicle, thereafter vaccinating from arm to arm. He vaccinated a number of children, including his own child and the child of General Herbin. Sometime after, smallpox broke out, and most of the vaccinated children were attacked, Dr. Defresne's and General Herbin's both dying of it." They rightly concluded that the vaccine had offered no protection and Defresne wrote a letter to the Vaccination Committee about it. They replied with asking for more particulars, and a series of questions Defresne did not respond to (likely because he had no heart for engaging in such "nonsensical subtleties"). He then reached out to Odier in Geneva, the great promoter of vaccination in Switzerland, who confirmed the fact that many of the other children had also died. His declaration was simply that "from what one father told him, he was far from certain that they did not all have spurious vaccine. (p. 262)"

I find it quite sad that in all the reasoning going on, no one even considered the possibility that: not only were the children who were previously inoculated (and died) clearly Not protected from disease, but the act of inoculation itself may have contributed to the disease process and increased the likelihood of dying from smallpox.

Eventually, the whole affair was forgotten, but similar conclusions were made in similar cases, like that of a little girl, whose father, Dr. Wolfram, was a regimental physician in the Prussian army. He wrote to Jenner to ensure the best matter for vaccination but when Jenner didn't reply he found other sources: the first of which did not take, but then lymph from another physician produced the vesicle on his daughter's arm which he described in full detail. Another example of one who followed as perfectly as he could have, the full, proper prescribed method of inoculation, yet, on the 13$^{th}$ of May, 1801, Dr. Wolfran's daughter died of smallpox (p. 263).

## Creating Cures or Creating Disease?

The enthusiasm for the "new protective" expanded to other diseases, besides smallpox. "De Carro found evidence at Constantinople that cowpox was an antidote also to the plague." "Struve believed that vaccination moderated the severity of scarlet fever, if it did not prevent the attack" and so did Careno. All these ideas about smallpox saving us from other diseases proved to be only theoretical and the few that were tested turned out to be obvious failures. One of the most notable was the effort to ward off the "sheep pox" in sheep through a vaccine. It failed so terribly, it was declared a clinical failure but also declared that the vaccine itself still "took" just like in a man. (meaning it caused eruptions etc.) As though that should still be something of value.

Jenner himself did not like these extensions in prophylaxis and as he states in a medical journal (p. 236), "I will just drop a hint – the vaccine disease, in my opinion, is not a preventive of the smallpox, but the smallpox itself." It was also claimed that "the country people of England, as well as the doctors, have represented the vaccine disease as the smallpox itself." Apparently, this is a breakthrough in medical science, to declare that "We have created the disease of smallpox through the inoculation of "cowpox!" It is hard for me to imagine that the "anti-vaccinists" were the only ones questioning the "victory" in such a declaration, though proof of this declaration was wanting.

It was this year, also, that M. Pasteur (I am supposing this is that same Louis Pasteur who helped to forever ingrain The Germ Theory of Disease into the brains of subsequent generations, as we'll discuss later) of The Academy of Science, helped to generalize the word, "Vaccine" so as to remove the "mystery" (of cowpox) and have it include a number of "protectives." This became the term later used to refer to a growing number and varying types of matter for the (so-called) preventive protection of all kinds of diseases, and is, of course, the term we use today. He also had his part in the (supposed) "scientific principle" for the "methodical attenuation of a virus."

## Objections Too Late

There were several who did voice their objections to the practice and claims of vaccination saying that there was too much "enthusiasm and authority" on the subject and not enough observable success or "experience" as well as a lack of scientific principles or as they put it, "disregard of the analytic method of Bacon, Locke and Condillac." Many years later, after the resurgence of smallpox, following bouts of Typhus, several objectors came forth to voice their frustrations. The "apologies" for cowpox not working, included claims that, if it did not irradicate smallpox, it at least caused milder forms. But it was pointed out, there did not exist milder forms since the cowpox invention than existed before it.

Doctors, like Dr. Carro (p. 234), "himself did, in fact see enough of cowpox ulceration on the arms to have made him doubt the mildness of the new protective, if not to have shown him what kind of pox it really was" (in other words, if there hadn't been the ready excuse about the type of pox, he likely would not have recanted how horrifically he originally viewed it). He also saw "enough of failure to protect from the smallpox to have satisfied him that the one kind of pox was altogether irrelevant to the other."

A few, anti-vaccinists, who were in opposition to the cowpox vaccination, and worth mentioning, are a Dr. Mosely, who wrote several treatises and essays on the subject, and a society of practical physicians who began a new series called, *The Medical Observer*, or *London Monthly Compendium of Medical Transactions*, and which became identified with the opposition to Cow-poxing, beginning in 1806 and continuing till 1811. Some reports demanded notice and stated plainly that, "the public had been misled by Jenner's famous doctrine of spurious cowpox in the cow, as if there were a true and a false cowpox." But, as Creighton points out, they were "too late." The damage had been done. As Creighton states, "They forgot that the whole of the early adverse evidence which ought to have stopped the delusion at the outset, had been overruled and explained away on that very plea as I have shown in previous chapters. The report concluded that "the security derived from vaccination, if not absolutely perfect, is as nearly so as can perhaps be expected from any human discovery." This report, on April 10th, 1807, was signed by a Sir Lucas Pepys, who submitted to having his grandson vaccinated by Jenner, though 2 years before he would as soon had his grandson bitten by a viper as vaccinated. Pepys is an example of the great change of opinion on the matter, due to the deceptiveness of Jenner and his theories and the growing acceptance by "great names" and "renowned physicians and societies." He played a significant part on its further acceptance and establishment of practice.

In following the qualms, silence, so called scrutiny and then unabashed acceptance of the new cowpox inoculation, in England, Germany and France, Dr, Creighton makes the well-deserved statement, "It becomes a matter of fresh interest to understand how this great nation, still breathing a spirit of scrutiny and rationalism, should have been hood-winked into adopting a medical dogma which had as little scientific basis in the pages of Jenner, as it had in the foolish heads of some Gloucestershire old women (p. 239). Here he is speaking particularly of the French, whose language had no corresponding word for Jenner's Variolae Vaccinae, (accepting it simply on good faith) but called it "smallpox of the cow" until it was simply changed to Vaccine.

The unnecessarily ulcerated arms, the deaths of countless infants, the ill health of untold thousands, if not millions (in this century alone)... all because a theory, that was never proven, became the accepted practice of a myriad of physicians, bowing to the perceived authority and professionalism of the Royal Academy and the growing popularity of Vaccination.

## Introducing Other Diseases

Besides the lack of protection, and mutilation from the inoculation, (as other physicians were pointing out in Gibb's book (p. 14) -including ones that still believed vaccines offered protection against smallpox!) there is the problem of relaying other infections, diseases, and adverse conditions due to vaccination. A group of French and American doctors who stalwartly held to the efficacy of vaccination against Smallpox admitted that "It is affirmed also, that other diseases are introduced into the system at the same time with the Cow-Pox." Among those, dwarfism seemed to be a result. Also, what they termed, "troublesome skin diseases." And in sad conclusion that, "children never enjoy good health after vaccination, however firm it may have been before."

A Professor Bartlett, who Gibbs calls a very "candid and able man" lectured at the University of New York on how Pulmonary Consumption was related to such practice. He showed data that over half of a group of vaccinated children had died later of Tubercular Consumption (Tuberculosis) (p. 14). Upon many other studies sighted, the consensus was that there were more deaths from tuberculosis among the vaccinated than death by other diseases. In other studies of vaccination (in later studies and for other diseases: including measles, rubella, hepatitis etc.) tuberculosis is a common aftermath of the vaccinated. I believe that the breaching of the cellular responses, through the delivery of toxins into the blood stream, our first lines of defense being compromised, what would have normally been a skin rash (or boils etc.) type of response to exposure of toxins or typical seasonal and epidemic diseases, becomes instead a disease affecting the lungs and other bodily organs, producing far more deadly consequences than the typical skin eruptions that would occur in one exposed naturally to disease.

Indeed, I believe you will find that among young children (with uncompromised immune systems) their first reaction to threatening toxins will be some sort of skin rash, accompanied by a fever. Children whose lymph systems have become too clogged will experience less cellular responses. 2nd level reactions to toxin overload will include "cold and flu symptoms": coughing, sneezing, congestion etc. As uncomfortable as these may be, they are all "normal" reactions of our bodily system to rid itself of "toxins" or foreign material (viral fractions, mold, smoke, putrid air and other sensitivities). Death and other serious issues, as organ damage: heart disease, respiratory collapse, lung disease, brain and CNS damage, occur only when a great many factors are compromised, poisoned or damaged at once. The more toxins you put into your body, the worse the damage potential. We will talk of this more later, but it is an observable fact from the earliest days of inoculating with diseased fragments (material).

Robert Alexander Gunn, in his book, Vaccination, Its Fallacies and Evils, says, "Even if there was any evidence to prove that vaccination was a prophylactic against small-pox, the appalling evils that have been and are still produced by it are sufficient to condemn the practice as a crime. Every physician of experience has met with numerous cases of cutaneous eruptions, erysipelas, and syphilis, which were directly traceable to vaccination, and if these could all be collected and presented in one report, they would form a more terrible picture than the worst that has ever been drawn to portray the horrors of small-pox (Gunn p. 21)."

It was right around this time, also that a new disease was becoming epidemic in Northern Italy. Italy had vaccination publicly enforced in 1806, and in subsequent years they began experiencing, what Dr. Creighton called Vaccinal Syphilis. A disease that is (supposedly) transmitted sexually, but became an epidemic so widespread, it could only be explained through some other mode of transfer. While no one seemed to want to blame the "golden child" of vaccination, it could hardly be explained any other way, than some contamination of the vaccines. Dr. Creighton wrote an entire book called, *Natural History of Cowpox and Syphilis*, which I have not been able to procure, but he mentions it in some detail in his book of *Jenner and Vaccination*. "I have entered into the evidence concerning these and other epidemics of the kind, and have stated the conclusion, which has not been as yet impugned, that the so-called syphilitic properties of the vaccine were not a contamination of it by another virus, but a revival, through carelessness as to over-ripeness, etc., of those inherent properties of cowpox to which it owed its original colloquial name of pox." In other words, it was not because of a random "contamination" of some vaccines but was a result of the original entities in the vaccine which, as part of their nature, was designed to cause disease.

I want to state briefly here that this is still a tactic used to sidestep the injurious nature of vaccines when the damage is so undeniably linked to them, to say it was a "contamination of a certain lot of vaccines" rather than admit the reality that all vaccines are, by their very nature, injurious. (we will also see this happen in the STORIES section of the triplets who all became autistic on the same day.)

## Assent to a Religious Belief?

We have already discussed the rise in diseases like tuberculosis in those who had been vaccinated. By 1840, people were growing discontent with the results of vaccination since the smallpox epidemics continued to return -particularly with bouts of typhus in between. Yet, throwing out the idea of vaccination and/or inoculation was not the resort, but rather a desire, by many, to go back to the "old methods" of inoculation. Dr. Creighton points out that the degree to which people held to the idea of vaccination, was of a continued religious fervor. As he writes, "In these debates nothing is more remarkable than the unanimous expression of belief that vaccine prevented smallpox; it was the real or religious assent to the most important of the several propositions of the complex doctrine."

During the 1880's there were cries for lessening the penalties, fines, and imprisonment for enforcing compulsory vaccination. A deputation to address these concerns was organized by the president of the Royal Society and consisted of himself and Professor Huxley, the president of the Royal College of physicians, the president of the Royal College of surgeons, the president of the General Medical Council and others. The president justified his actions by claiming that, "noncompliance with the vaccination law appeared to "trench closely upon the application, at least, of a scientific principle." When asked by a correspondent to state what was the scientific principle, the president of the Royal Society stated briefly, "the principle to which I referred was that of vaccination." Such circular reasoning, which fails, at every turn, to adequately question the validity of vaccination itself, and uses vaccination, to validate vaccination, is, indeed akin to an outlandish religious fervor.

## Saving Face Vs Saving Humanity

By 1818, vaccination stood in great need of some excuse for failure, as the continuation of cases was hard to ignore. The "ingenious doctrine" of "modified smallpox" erupted. The epidemic of 1817-1818, Creighton declares, was, perhaps the greatest moment of hesitation for many in the profession, and they seemed inclined to agree with many of the common people that there was something very wrong with Jenner's teaching. I will take the following directly from Creighton's book on the matter, "However painful, yet it is a duty we owe to the public and the profession to apprise them that the number of all ranks suffering under smallpox, who have previously undergone vaccination by the most skillful practitioners is at present surprisingly great. The subject is so serious and so deeply involves the dearest interests of humanity as well as those of the medical character, that we shall not fail in directing our utmost attention to it. Unhappily, the dearest interests of humanity had to give way before the dearest interests of the medical character. The credit of the profession was at stake. A surrender in Jenner's lifetime would have been too humiliating seeing that parliament had been induced to vote him 10,000 pounds in 1802 and 20,000 pounds in 1807 upon the warrant of medical evidence." Creighton (p. 183), "It is hard to believe that the many educated and conscientious men, who belonged to the medical profession of Britain in those years, had given their reasoned consent to a doctrine and practice so full of frauds and fallacies that a later generation will hardly bear to have the naked facts exhibited to the public gaze." Indeed, the facts appeared, at times, to be so insanely riveted with failures and injury, to reveal it all would've been a great embarrassment, to say the least.

## The Only "Cure"

So disappointing that the ideas of more nutrition, a cleaner environment, rigorous play in the outside air and sunshine, or a great number of things truly conducive to health could not have been the focus during this era. Creighton mentions a Lord

Shaftsbury, as the “only person who showed a nidus of what smallpox was really about”, and who remarked during a debate that, “smallpox was chiefly confined to the lowest class of the population, and he believed that with improved lodging-houses, the disease might be all but exterminated.”

If only this could have been the advice that was followed by the public. But we have not yet discussed the greatest proof for the failure of vaccination.

# CHAPTER 2

## DATA DOESN'T LIE

There truly is a dizzying amount of implications for the failure of Vaccines (and inoculation) and the responses and excuses and exchange (and change) of terms to continually avert straightforward and simple scientific scrutiny, so that the battle of the efficacy of the pox vaccine became more a battle over terms, methods of vaccinating, timing, types of eruptions etc. and little about proving what I would state as the **only good things** vaccination could have to offer, namely, improvement of the immune system and/or protection from future disease. **Neither of which were proven experimentally or scientifically**.

Perhaps the greatest way to prove its failure or success is to see how mass vaccination in a country or province, affects its population following its enforcement. So, does getting more people vaccinated lower the death rate from these diseases than years of non-enforcement during or following epidemics?? Let's look at the data.

Data both by Dr. Creighton and George Gibbs (another "anti-vaxer" who wrote, *The Evils of Vaccination, with a Protest Against Its Legal Enforcement)* and a few others show, specifically, that death rates from smallpox were considerably higher in the year following a compulsory law (where everyone was demanded to be vaccinated under penalty of law and fined for not complying). One of the years this was most severe was 1853.

Dr. Creighton points out the fact that in places like Germany and England (where more acclaim to the "grand discovery" of vaccination led to a continual downplay of its clear failure), the numbers may have been far less than accurate. Yet, even then, failure can be seen significantly. "Nearly 125,000 deaths in Prussia from 1871-1872 in lists kept by the police there. It was Not among the unvaccinated that the greatest casualties of the epidemic took place (Creighton p. 351)." In Bavaria, cases of smallpox, recorded by the Bureau of statistics in Munich were 30,742 of which the vaccinated made up 95.7% (29,429) and the unvaccinated 4.3% (1,313). These included 3,994 recorded deaths among the vaccinated and 790 of unvaccinated (743 of which were infants).

George Gibbs records similar and even more frequent deaths, in his concise book: *The Evils of Vaccination, with a Protest Against its Legal Enforcement.* He gives tables that show the increase and decreases of death by smallpox, particularly following the year it was a major epidemic in London and several other places around the world: 1838. While we see a huge decrease the following year, subsequent years show both increases and decreases each subsequent year, until you reach the 1850's where deaths climb to staggering heights virtually unseen before. Gibbs is making his plea against the Compulsory Vaccination act of 1853. He quotes physicians who have seen so many injuries of various types including deaths in their practices that they abandoned the practice altogether. Yet, in Gibb's day a decree was being set forth with government power and authority to demand the vaccination of all (particularly all the children) of England. I will mention just a few of the examples he records.

"The parent or guardian of every child (up to 13 yrs. of age), on or after the 1st day of January 1857, who shall not already have been successfully vaccinated, nor had the Small-Pox, shall, within four calendar months, bring the child to the public vaccinator for the purpose of being vaccinated (Gibbs p. 7)."

"It shall be lawful for the managing committees of schools receiving aid from government grants, the masters of workhouses, and keepers of prisons, to inquire into the vaccination of children attending such schools, or of the inmates of such workhouses, asylums or prisons, respectively, and to direct the vaccination of all such persons therein as they find unvaccinated."

I am quoting a mere 2 of 24 such decrees, and the penalty for guardians was up to 20 shillings and up to 5 shillings each day after for every day of non-compliance. Obstructing anyone employed in the execution of this act or those who violated ANY regulation or direction of the General Board of Health, were liable to a penalty of up to 5 Pounds.

George Gibbs goes on to sight the many persons who objected to the practice, and I quote, "First are those [who object to the practice of vaccination,] who regard the introduction of a disease into the system, under the pretense of keeping it healthy in futurity, or, indeed, under any pretense whatever, not merely as a gross absurdity, but as a direct violation of the Law of God; for if the soul's health be the primary object of care, the blessed gift of bodily health is surely not to be treated with contempt. But there are others who object to vaccination on the ground that it is not what it pretends to be [IE] a protection against Small-Pox. They say that a glance at the varying mortality from this disorder in successive years is sufficient to prove this proposition."

protection against Small-Pox. They say that a glance at the varying mortality from this disorder in successive years is sufficient to prove this proposition. For instance, the deaths in London from Small-Pox were,—

| Year | | Deaths | Year | | Deaths |
|---|---|---|---|---|---|
| In 1838* | ... | 3817 | In 1845 | ... | 909 |
| „ 1839 | ... | 634 | „ 1846 | ... | 257 |
| „ 1840 | ... | 1235 | „ 1847 | .. | 955 |
| „ 1841 | ... | 1053 | „ 1848 | ... | 1617 |
| „ 1842 | ... | 360 | „ 1849 | ... | 518 |
| „ 1843 | ... | 438 | „ 1850 | ... | 498 |
| „ 1844 | ... | 1804 | „ 1851 | ... | 1066 |

* In this year Small-Pox was *epidemic* in London, and generally throughout England.

A 3

He goes on to sight a chart (p. 9) showing the deaths from smallpox in London from 1838-1851 which began with over 3,000 (the year it was epidemic) and rises and falls each year thereafter, never exceeding less than 2,000. The death rates in all England and Wales fluctuated similarly. Besides that, returns to a Small-Pox hospital showed that out of over 4,055 patients, 2,167 (or more than half) had been vaccinated (p.10). A physician in London at a Small-Pox hospital for 50 years relayed that out of 298 vaccinated patients admitted in 1838 at least 31 died. A story in The Lancet, Jan. 1853, tells of a pregnant woman who had been vaccinated as an infant and had been revaccinated (by the physician documenting the story). A few days after, he was called, hurriedly, to see the patient who had developed intense pain in her loins, had an eruption on the third day, and her throat was so inflamed she could hardly swallow. She aborted the baby and had a large amount of hemorrhaging. The eruption showed two large vesicles as you would expect to find on someone newly vaccinated. She died in just 6 days (p.10-11).

These are just a few of the reported data, and stories that become a repeated problem throughout this time. A Biographer relays his observations on the reality of Small-Pox saying that "it was an Epidemic Disease over 50 years ago and a long time before that, and that it was kept in existence through the practice of inoculation; and that its fatality was fearfully increased by the barbarous method of treatment (p.11). Also, that the mode of dealing with such a disorder was as opposite as could be imagined to the "dictates of nature or to common sense"!

The following table shows the result of this rigid enforcement in a proportionate mortality very much greater than in this country, and in some instances twice as great :—

| Town or Country. | Year. | Population. | | Deaths. | | Proportion per 1000. |
|---|---|---|---|---|---|---|
| London ............... | 1851 | 2,373,799 | ... | 55,254 | ... | 23·3 |
| England and Wales... | " | 17,922,768 | ... | 395,933 | ... | 22 |
| Liverpool............... | 1850 | 258,236 | ... | 7,500 | ... | 29 |
| Manchester ............ | " | 228,433 | ... | 6,680 | ... | 29 |
| Birmingham ......... | " | 173,951 | ... | 4,056 | ... | 23·3 |
| Leeds ................. | " | 101,343 | ... | 2,502 | ... | 24·6 |
| Dublin.................. | 1851 | 258,361 | ... | 6,931 | ... | 26·8 |
| Cork .................. | " | 85,745 | ... | 2,002 | ... | 23·3 |
| Limerick .............. | " | 53,448 | ... | 1,418 | ... | 26·5 |
| Galway .............. | " | 34,057 | ... | 789 | ... | 23 |

* *Epidem. Society's Report*, p. 6.

13

| Town or Country | Year. | Population. | | Deaths. | | Proportion per 1000. |
|---|---|---|---|---|---|---|
| Lower Austria......... | 1850 | 1,538,047 | ... | 54,970 | ... | 35·7 |
| Upper Austria......... | " | 852,323 | ... | 23,646 | ... | 27·7 |
| Styria .................. | " | 1,006,971 | ... | 30,534 | ... | 30·3 |
| Illyria .................. | " | 738,180 | ... | 34,630 | ... | 46·9 |
| Trieste.................. | " | 82,597 | ... | 3,283 | ... | 39·7 |
| Tyrol .................. | " | 859,706 | ... | 25,276 | ... | 29·4 |
| Bohemia .............. | " | 4,409,900 | ... | 170,432 | ... | 38·6 |
| Moravia .............. | " | 1,799,838 | ... | 55,637 | ... | 30·9 |
| Silesia .................. | " | 438,516 | ... | 12,123 | ... | 27·6 |
| Gallicia .............. | " | 4,555,477 | ... | 140,329 | ... | 30·8 |
| Bukowina ........... | " | 380,826 | ... | 11,070 | ... | 29.0 |
| Dalmatia............... | " | 393,715 | ... | 9,442 | ... | 23.9 |
| Lombardy ........... | " | 2,725,740 | ... | 92,550 | ... | 33·9 |
| Venice .................. | " | 2,281,732 | ... | 76,150 | ... | 33·3 |
| Military Frontiers without the seven Burghs. ............ | " | 1,009,109 | ... | 44,610* | ... | 44·2 |

Notice how the number of deaths in London soar (from just over 1,000) to over 55,000 the year following vaccine mandate? Over 55 times higher! Gibbs goes on to show tables of death rates in countries all around the globe from Smallpox. Over and over, we see the mortality rates far higher in countries where vaccination was enforced, usually at least twice as high. (I share some more graphs in the SCIENCE chapter which are also worth noting.)

Where then, is the scientific proof? Where is the protection, finally achieved, that might justify the years of inoculation progressing into vaccination? The years of proliferating and spreading volumes of diseased material, "perfecting" the method, the use of thousands and tens of thousands of individuals used as specimens? The destruction or compromise (great and small) of so many immune systems, and even lives. Where are the results that finally proved it was all worthwhile? Oh, what a service they would have rendered to the world and future generations, if only there would have been the moral fortitude and dedication to the truth, to swallow the pride and expense for the sake of their fellow brethren and, indeed, humanity itself! Yet, they never could have imagined the world of evil they failed to extinguish or how broad and how long it would be perpetuated in the world.

The works I have mentioned here are certainly not the entire history, but I hope I have given enough information and data to convince you of the inefficacy of the cow pox vaccination. If not, I invite you to read the books available on the subject (from the anti-vaxer's point of view) and hear their cries of insurrection and pleading for yourself. I know some of those resources may be hard to come by and I am hoping they will become more readily available.

**In conclusion**:

Jenner's experiments and declarations were certainly NOT in line with scientific principles or methods. There is proof throughout Creighton's observations that he purposely favored some subjects while dismissing others. Sometimes he favored older subjects (who were less likely to react as they had already been exposed to the pox). With all the conjecture of what vaccination was supposed to accomplish, there never was any actual, scientific or consistent proof that vaccination provided any protection against smallpox, whatever. In fact, the opposite is the reality, especially when you observe its effects on a nation or province. The practice of vaccination did more to introduce toxins into the body than otherwise would've existed, and perpetuated disease both in cows (and horses) and people through the practice of proliferation of diseased tissue (for collection of matter to inoculate) as well as perpetuate the disease of smallpox itself to be more abundant and persist longer than it ever would have if things had been left to their natural course, but especially if measures would've been taken to eradicate, instead of perpetuate the disease in the first place: like separating the diseased cow from the heard, or better understanding of cleanliness and improved living conditions.

These, in truth, are the real deliverers from the smallpox epidemics, as very few of that era were pointing out.

I believe it highly worth mentioning that there was a great effort during this time to eradicate from the earth all future epidemics and even memory of smallpox. Suffice it to say, it did not happen. Yet, the medical establishment declares that "the smallpox vaccine, created by Edward Jenner in 1796, was the first successful vaccine to be developed." That, "He observed that milkmaids who previously had caught cowpox did not catch smallpox and showed that a similar inoculation could be used to prevent smallpox in other people." They also say, "The World Health Organization launched an intensified plan to eradicate smallpox in 1967. Widespread immunization and surveillance were conducted around the world for several years. [They also say] The last known natural case was in Somalia in 1977. In 1980 WHO declared smallpox eradicated - the only infectious disease to achieve this distinction. This remains among the most notable and profound public health successes in history." Does it, indeed?

Again, as with so many other "viral diseases" that are now vaccinated against, I would ask: what are the disease symptoms that are, supposedly, non-existent now? What sort of "pox sores" that could be observed then, never show up? (I'll talk more about this idea in later chapters.) Does that mean that the sores cows get on their udders, termed cowpox have also been irradicated? I hope so, but if that is the case it is because we now have rules of cleanliness concerning our milked cows that didn't exist then.

The truth remains that the smallpox declaration, as one of the greatest human achievements, became the catalyst for one of the most profoundly disastrous consequences in human history. The damage that has been done to countless human lives, and especially infants and children, is one of the most remarkably insidious evils that continues to plague our modern medical establishments.

While doing this study, I must say that one thing consistently jumped out at me, and that is the reality that even though this vaccine history is nearly (or over, depending on how one looks at it) 200 years ago, the pattern we see emerging, the methods used, the excuses given, the data overlooked or altogether disregarded, the blind acceptance due to perceived authorities and experts on the matter and the confusion produced by changing the terms or language, or what constitutes "successful" vaccines, reflects, so exquisitely, the way vaccination exists and is administered today. Only, they have better succeeded rewriting the narrative and hiding the truth.

Before moving on to other voices on the subject, I want to share Dr. Creighton's conclusion in his own words:

"The task which I set before me when I began this book was to explain to myself how the medical profession, in various countries, could have come to fall under the enchantment of an illusion. I believe that they were misled most of all by the name of "smallpox of the cow" under which the new protective was first brought to their notice for that grand initial error, blameworthy in its inception and still more so in the furtive manner of its publication, the sole responsibility rests with Jenner. The profession as a whole, has been committed before now to erroneous doctrines and injurious practices which have been upheld by its solid authority for generations. Lesage's satire upon bloodletting, in *Gil Blas* which appeared in 1715, aught of itself to have made that practice ludicrous in the eyes of the world, but bloodletting survived 100 years after that in all countries, and in the country of Sangrado, it survived 150 years. The apology for it or explanation of this abandonment which was still being taught in lectures 20 years ago was that diseases had changed their type from sthenic to asthenic and that in our asthenic age bloodletting was no longer necessary. It is difficult to conceive what will be the excuse made for a century of cowpoxing; but it cannot be doubted that the practice will appear in as absurd a light to the common sense of the 20th century as bloodletting now does to us. Vaccination differs, however, from all previous errors of the faculty, in being maintained as the law of the land on the warrant of medical authority."

**If only vaccination were as absurd to us, now, as the past barbarous practice of bloodletting!**

I don't want to spend too much time in this history period alone, as it could take, literally, volumes of books, and one could still make the argument that the vaccines of today are not as they began. This may be quite true. I would make the argument that they have become much worse.

## Words Against Vaccines Throughout History

### From Physicians and Scientists

Here are some quotes from several others who have, through the ages, shared, all along, their unanimous stance on the great deception and disaster of vaccination. These are some of the voices and cries that should have been heeded long ago. It is fitting to give them a place in this book to remember them and realize that those who take the anti-vaccinist stance are far from alone.

19TH CENTURY (1800s)

"There does not exist one single fact, in all the experiments and improvements made in science, which can support the idea of vaccination. A vaccinated people will always be a sickly people, short lived and degenerate." —Dr. Alexander Wilder, MD, "Vaccination: A Medical Fallacy", editor of the New York Medical Tribune, 1879

"I have seen leprosy and syphilis communicated by vaccination. Leprosy is becoming very common in Trinidad; its increase being coincident with vaccination." —Dr. Hall Bakewell, Vaccinator General of Trinidad, 1868

"Cancer is reported to be increasing not only in England and the Continent, but in all parts of the world where vaccination is practised." —Dr. William S. Tebb, MA, MD, DPH, "The Increase of Cancer", 1892

"Leprosy arose with vaccination." —Sir Ronald Martin, MD, 1868

"Syphilis has undoubtedly been transmitted by vaccination." —Sir William Osler Bt., MD, FRS, FRCP

"To no medium of transmission is the widespread dissemination of this class of disease (syphilis) so largely indebted as to Vaccination." —Dr. B.F. Cornell, MD, 1868

"Every intelligent person who takes the time to investigate vaccination, will find abundant evidence in the published writings and public records of the advocates of vaccination, to prove its utter worthlessness, without reading a line of antivaccination literature. And if we could add to this all the suppressed facts, we would have a mass of evidence before which no vaccinator would dare to hold up his head."—Dr. Robert A. Gunn, MD, "Vaccination: Its Fallacies and Evils", 1882

"I have no faith in vaccination, nay, I look upon it with greatest disgust and firmly believe that it is often the medium of conveying many filthy and loathsome diseases from one child to another, and it is no protection from smallpox." —Dr. William Collins, MD, London, 1882

"Vaccination has made murder legal. Vaccination does not protect against smallpox, but is followed by blindness and scrofula. Jennerism is the most colossal humbug which the human race has been burdened with by FRAUD and DECEIT." —Mr. Mitchell, member of the British House of Commons

"Of these dogmas, I believe the practice known as vaccination to be the most absurd and most pernicious. I do not believe that a single person has ever been protected from smallpox by it; while I know that many serious bodily evils and even deaths, have resulted from its employment. The whole theory is founded upon assumption, contrary to common sense and entirely opposed to all known principles of physiology. Every physician of experience, has met with numerous cases of cutaneous eruptions, erysipelas and syphilis, which were directly traceable to vaccination, and if these cases could be collected and presented in one report, they would form a more terrible picture than the worst that has ever been drawn of the horrors of smallpox." —Dr. Robert A. Gunn, MD, Dean of the United States Medical College of New York

"Vaccination is a monstrosity, a misbegotten offspring of error and ignorance; and, being such, it should have no place in either hygiene or medicine... Believe not in vaccination, it is a worldwide delusion, an unscientific practice, a fatal superstition with consequences measured today by tears and sorrow without end." —Dr. Carlo Ruta, Professor of Materia Medica at the University of Perugia, Italy, 1896

"Vaccination is a gigantic delusion. It has never saved a single life. It has been the cause of so much disease, so many deaths, such a vast amount of utterly needless and altogether undeserved suffering, that it will be classed by the coming generation among the greatest errors of an ignorant and prejudiced age, and its penal enforcement the foulest blot." —Alfred R. Wallace, LLD DUBL., DCL OXON., FRS, etc., 1898

20TH CENTURY (1900s)

"The great epidemics of deadly diseases, in animals and mankind, are caused by vaccination." —Charles M. Higgins, "The Horrors of Vaccination: Exposed and Illustrated", 1920

"l believe vaccination has been the greatest delusion that has ensnared mankind in the last three centuries. It originated in FRAUD, ignorance and error. It is unscientific and impracticable. It has been promotive of very great evil, and I cannot accredit it any good." —Dr. R. K. Noyse, MD, Resident Surgeon of the Boston City Hospital, "Self Curability of Disease"

"The chief, if not the sole, cause of the monstrous increase in cancer has been vaccination." —Dr. Robert Bell; Vice President, International Society for Cancer Research, British Cancer Hospital, 1922

"Vaccination is the most outrageous insult that can be offered to any pure minded man or woman. It is the boldest and most impious attempt to mar the works of God that has been attempted for ages. The stupid blunder of doctorcraft has wrought all the evil that it ought, and it is time that free American citizens arise in their might and blot out the whole blood poisoning business." — Dr. J.M. Peebles, MD, MA, PhD, "Vaccination: A Curse and Menace to Personal Liberty", 1900

"Cancer was practically unknown until the cowpox vaccination began to be introduced. I have seen 200 cases of cancer and never saw a case in an unvaccinated person." —Dr. W.B. Clark, MD, Indiana, New York Times article, 1909

"At present, intelligent people do not have their children vaccinated, nor does the law now compel them to. The result is not, as the Jennerians prophesied, the extermination of the human race by smallpox; on the contrary more people are now killed by vaccination than by smallpox." —George Bernard Shaw, 1944

"The English Ministry of Health omits to state that in 1872, when 85% of the infants born were vaccinated, there were 19,000 deaths from smallpox in England and Wales. While in 1925, when less than half the children born were vaccinated, there were only 6 deaths from that disease." —Dr. Eleanor McBean, PhD, ND, "The Poisoned Needle", 1957

"Vaccination causes miscarriage. A careful check showed that 47% of women who had been vaccinated in the second or third month of pregnancy, failed to give birth to a normal child." — "Vaccination at Work", The Consulting Pediatrician of Lanarkshire County Council, The Lancet (London), p.47, December 6, 1952

"My honest opinion is that vaccine is the cause of more disease and suffering than anything I could name." —Dr. Harry R. Bybee

"Vaccination, instead of being the promised blessing to the world, has proved to be a curse of such sweeping devastation that it has caused more death and disease than war, pestilence, and plague combined. There is no scourge (with the possible exception of atomic radiation) that is more destructive to our nation's health than this monument of human deception—this slayer of the innocent— this crippler of body and brain—the poisoned needle." —Dr. Eleanor McBean, PhD, ND, "The Poisoned Needle", 1957

"The greatest LIE ever told is that vaccines are safe and effective."—Dr. Leonard Horowitz, MPH (Master of Public Health), DMD, MA, Harvard University graduate

21ST CENTURY (2000s)

"The entire vaccine program is based on massive FRAUD."—Dr. Russell L. Blaylock, M.D., neurosurgeon, editorial staff of Journal of American Physicians and Surgeons

"Vaccinations do not work. They don't work at all." —Dr. Lorraine Day, MD

"Vaccinations are now carried out for purely commercial reasons because they fetch huge profits for the pharmaceutical industry. There is no scientific evidence that vaccinations are of any benefit." —Dr. Gerhard Buchwald, MD,

"Vaccination: A business based on FEAR" "Don't get your flu shot." —Dr. Raymond Francis, D.Sc., M.Sc., RNC, chemist, MIT graduate

"My own personal view is that vaccines are unsafe and WORTHLESS. I will not allow myself to be vaccinated again. Vaccines may be profitable but in my view, they are neither safe nor effective." –Dr. Vernon Coleman, MB, ChB, DSc (Hon)

"Everyone who is vaccinated is vaccine injured—whether it shows up right away or later in life." —Dr. Shiv Chopra, B.V.S., A.H., M.Sc., PhD, Fellow of the World Health Organization, former senior scientist at Health Canada

"Vaccines are the backbone of the entire Pharmaceutical Industry. If they can make these children sick from a very early age, they become customers for life. The money isn't really to be made in the vaccine industry. The money is made by Big Pharma with all of the drugs that are given to treat and address all of the illnesses that are subsequent to the side effects of vaccines."—Dr. Sherri Tenpenny, D.O. (osteopathic medical doctor)

"Studies are increasingly pointing to the conclusion that vaccines represent a dangerous assault to the immune system leading to autoimmune diseases like Multiple Sclerosis, Lupus, Juvenile Onset Diabetes, Fibromyalgia, and Cystic Fibrosis, as well as previously rare disorders like brain cancer, SIDS (Sudden Infant Death Syndrome), childhood leukemia, autism, and asthma."—Dr. Zoltan Rona, MD, "Natural Alternatives to Vaccination"

"The vaccine industry is itself a FRAUD. I spent my whole career studying vaccines."—Dr. Shiv Chopra, B.V.S., A.H., M.Sc., Ph.D., Fellow of the World Health Organization, "Corrupt to the Core"

Truly, the only thing more concrete than such unanimous historical consensus (of which this is a small portion) about vaccines are the stories of those who have experienced firsthand its devastation, which we will hear next.

# CHAPTER 3

## LISTEN TO THE STORIES

I want to insert a few stories of actual damage from vaccines, before moving on. I also want to include them JUST AS WRITTEN, without modifying the way the stories were originally shared. Although this is only a fraction of true stories that exist, I will share a few here and more in the chapter VACCINES AND THEIR INGREDIENTS and in the appendix section: MORE STORIES. The stories begin with those from my own circle of friends and move on to those shared from a public platform. Most are shared with permission, and I have only included details that the authors and/or sharers have included. There are many more to be found, and I will include sites and links in the appendix section where they can be found, along with many more.

It is strange how certain realities can seem so obvious to one, looking on with an open mind and willingness to see the truth staring them in the face, and yet becomes apparently hidden from those with a clear agenda and eyes only willing to see success and confirmation of one's own ideas and proposals. In the area of vaccination, though, it has been a common belief and continuously upheld practice in medical schools and establishments, to the point which shields it from any power of scrutiny and often silences the voices that would otherwise cry out. Yet, even still, these voices continue to cry out, because the damage is so staggering and heart breaking. I record these stories here, partly because they deserve to be remembered.

In my own circle I know, personally, many parents who saw adverse reactions of all kinds after their children were vaccinated. Just to mention a few, and whose names I'll not mention (unless permission has been granted to do so): One friend of mine whose son who was vaccinated at an early age, felt they lost at least two years of development after he was vaccinated and he experienced various other side effects much later including cancer.  Another mother relayed how in horror she watched her daughter (in her teens) slip into a kind of coma and feared she had "lost her"  (this was on the medical table right after her vaccine) until her body did at last recover, and she slowly regained function again. Another mom, after dutiful research and observation, believed the vaccines her daughters received were the cause of their chronic and very painful nervous system disorder (they call it CRPS), which made them feel as though their limbs were on fire!

Another mother watched her son develop autism and saw his entire personality change: he lost language skills, had to be taught how to play, screamed for large portions of the day and suffered episodes of violence, while at other times he would stare into space for hours at a time.  He also suffered with digestion issues and chronic diarrhea. His family wondered whether he would ever be normal enough to graduate school or have any sort of normal life. This story does have a happy ending, for after many tears, much prayer and labors of love, he was able to regain his brain function and the violent episodes subsided. He regained his ability to speak, communicate and regulate his emotions. He has spent years creating his own you tube channel, and he now works for a film making company. I know this young man, personally. His name is Jackson, and his story is quite an inspiring one. His mother is currently writing a book that contains the testimony of their tumultuous yet beautiful journey. I hope it will reach many other moms and families and give them hope.

Another mother (whom I know) shares how her daughter, Jodie, experienced her first seizure at 11 mo. old after receiving her first round of vaccines. She has since had episodes that have included up to 100 seizures in a single day and been in 3 comas. Her life with her daughter has been a continual challenge. Efforts in dietary changes and special care have brought her slowly from 90 lbs. to now well over a hundred and slowed the number and duration of seizures. As many know, who have experienced the aftermath of vaccine poison, neurological and personality changes are a repeated problem and one of the most devastating. For those who have experienced severe trauma, there is always hope that healing is possible, but often it does not happen.

One more story I'll mention from a friend.

Dawson was a perfectly healthy little boy. His mother described him as kind, smart and actively engaged in learning. They avoided any vaccines from the time he was 1 yr. to 5 yrs. old. Before attending Kindergarten, he received several doses of vaccines to "catch him up" to the CDC's schedule. After that time, his mom noticed several sudden and undeniable changes, both in his personality and his health. He developed extreme food allergies causing him to projectile vomit and lose a lot of weight. She said he looked pale with purple bags around his eyes. He used multiple inhalers for asthma and had his tonsils and adenoids removed in an attempt to combat the hyperactivity, bed-wetting and other related issues. Worst of all, his personality changed and he became violent towards other children and even constructed a suicide plan after being moved to another school.

Only moms who have had to deal with the horror and drama (and guilt) of these sorts of changes to their children can truly relate to the emotional toil such episodes bring on the families doing their best to try to deal with the aftermath of vaccine poisoning. In this case, as with multitudes of others, putting the pieces together, trying to find healing and understanding the cause didn't come till much later.

There are very many, lesser extreme, stories of children who simply underwent what seemed like extremely long bouts of cold and flu. Sickness to the point of not being able to function in normal activities, including play, often for months at a time. Some with personality changes less severe but noticed by their closest care-givers. There are others, like Katie. A friend of mine who never realized she was vaccine damaged until genetic testing showed that vaccine damage was responsible for her many allergies and auto-immune disorders. Then there are, of course, those who seem to experience no issues at all. These are the lucky ones. Not all stories end so well, and some don't experience issues until later. In every case, the greater the number of vaccines, the greater and more extreme the damage.

Those who suffer the highest death rates from vaccines are, undoubtedly, babies. The number of infant deaths from vaccines, alone, is so staggering, (millions upon millions) that, if this death toll were known to the public, one could hardly find a reason to excuse its use, even if it did deliver the protection manufacturers claimed (a protection never proven). The reality of vaccine damage is so widespread that it can hardly be kept in the dark anymore. Just in my own small sphere, I have many stories of vaccine injury I could tell and yet, amazingly, or rather unbelievably, you can NOT find ONE SINGLE STORY online about victims damaged by vaccines on Google or You Tube (unless you know exactly where to look). There are stories that pop up on FB (if you follow those who share). There are whole websites dedicated to sharing stories and information about vaccines and vaccine damage (you'll find many in the Appendix). Some of these sites are hard to find, and there are stories shared as little as one year ago (or less), that have since disappeared or been redirected. For those that do exist, I have to have an exact story, or name, or web address to be able to find what I'm looking for, for if I type in anything about vaccines, their history, or damage caused by vaccines, all I will encounter is the familiar-sounding rhetoric of the importance of vaccination and its safety, etc. How is that possible? We live in an age where information is so available it's overwhelming. How is it that in this area all qualms on this subject matter are hushed? Buried. Unavailable. There's a reason why. There is a narrative being heavily propagated and tightly controlled, to eliminate as much information against vaccines, and pharmaceuticals as possible. They want people to forget its dark history so they can continue their agenda of vaccinating as much of the population as possible.

I am not exaggerating in the slightest, when I tell you that there are literally multitudes (in the millions at least) of stories and posts and claims and proofs of vaccine damage that have been scrubbed from internet history, and many that were simply not told. There are still stories that will make it through, particularly the extreme ones, because parents who have seen the worst sort of damage to their children, which can be explained no other way possible but by vaccines, the correlation being so obvious and immediate, that these voices are very hard, if not impossible, to drown out entirely.

Let me name a few:

This is a story of three triplets: Richie, Clair and Robbie and what happened to them in 2018. I will share a link to the FB post and video in the appendix.

Originally from the VAXXED documentary.

(See links in the Appendix sect.)

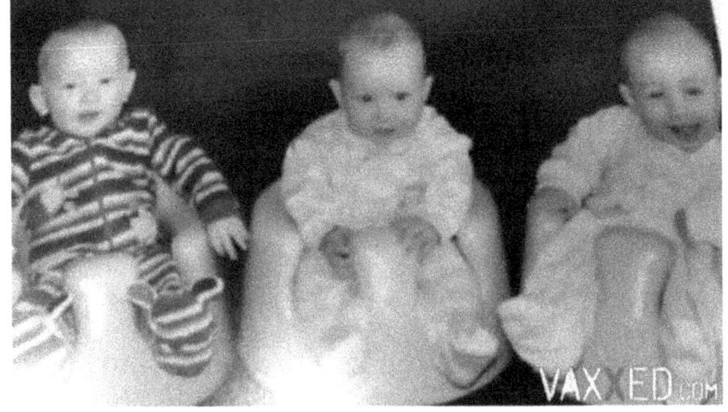


Brenda and David McDowell took their three healthy children in at 9 months old for a Pneumococcal vaccine. They share video footage of their three adorable triplets, smiling, happy and giggling at each other. The same day they received their vaccination shots, they drastically changed, never to be the same again. Just two hours later, Claire, their little girl "completely shut off" (their words) "as if she were blind and deaf. She just stared at the ceiling."

"At 2 pm Richie shut off. By the end of the day, Robbie looked like he was hit by a bus, he had a stunned look on his face." These three sweet babies, though not killed, lost a quality of life that would never return to them, and would leave their parents forever stunned and heart broken. The giggles stopped.

The smiling, babbling, furniture walking, even blinking, yawning, and sneezing stopped. They never held hands again. They never looked at each other again.

As a mom who adores my littles (now almost 3 yrs and 6 months) and loves to see the facial expressions, the eye contact, the little mouths babbling and making cooing sounds, the adorable smile and laugh of my baby that moves me to joy beyond words, I can't even imagine having that all taken away because I unwittingly allowed a doctor, who should've known better, to inject poison into my precious children. There is nothing on planet earth more heart-wrenching than that!

The McDowells found out about vaccine Injury Court about 5 years later, but by then it was too late to apply. They have spent hundreds of thousands of dollars trying to recover and heal their children. Seven Years after that horrid day, they found information saying that particular lot was, supposedly recalled for contamination, as it had already killed a 2 year old. All of it was hidden from the public.

The geneticist that they consulted said it is an "Impossibility" that three siblings get autism on the same day. That's not how genetics operates, and there is literally NO WAY for that to happen, genetically.

This is one of many that is so obvious, that to say damage did not happen from a vaccine, is literally insane. That it is all a coincidence, is beyond denial. This is Evil of the most extreme and vile kind, built on one of the greatest lies, somehow believed by millions... no, billions. This is one of the few stories that has not been successfully (at least not thoroughly) silenced.

## Attempts at Silencing

When I search the name, Nick Catone, what I find is a name to a gym, owned by a father who lost his child at 20 mo. of age (the reason is never explained, or even mentioned) and he runs this gym in honor of his, now deceased, son.

I had to do quite a bit of digging to find a news report that at least acknowledged his plight. From News12 New Jersey:

"A former professional fighter from New Jersey says that vaccines are to blame for the death of his son. Nick Catone is preparing to open a new gym in Ocean County next week. But he says while he is preparing for that, he is also preparing to take on the government over the unexpected death of his son 15 months ago.

Catone says that his son Nicholas was only 20 months old. He says the boy went to bed one night and did not wake up the next morning. This was May 12, 2017.

An autopsy report found that nothing was wrong. But Catone and his wife Marjorie did not find that acceptable. "Instantly I had this gut motherly instinct that the only thing that came across his path was that he was recently vaccinated," Marjorie Catone says.

Marjorie has been a nurse for 12 years. She says that she pulled her son's medical records to look for patterns and noticed that he kept getting sick after being vaccinated.

The Catones are taking their case to vaccine court. It is a low-profile program that compensates families who can prove that their child was injured or died because of vaccines.

"Brian Hooker lost his case in vaccine court 20 years ago. His son had autism." The Catones stated.

"After the vaccination, after his fever spiked, he then very quickly lost all language. He lost all eye contact. He lost any type of joint attention," Hooker says.

But pediatrician Mark Sawyer tells News 12 New Jersey that while side effects from vaccines are possible, their benefits are much greater than their risks.

The Catones say that they want to see changes in legislation.

"You get angry because it all could have been prevented. Nobody ever mentioned any of this to us," Nick Catone says.

Nick Catone's new 31,000-square-foot gym is a tribute to his son. It will open Sept. 8.

"This has been a dream of mine. It's gonna be hard to 100% enjoy it because I don't have my son. But I know he would want me to keep going," Catone says.

The Catone's say that a date for vaccine court has not yet been set."

This was written, Aug 30, 2018

This is one of Nick Catone's more recent posts about his own son: (excuse the language, but it's totally understandable)

"April 23rd, it was two days before you had your "Well Visit" and received the D-tap vaccine. You were so happy playing with Madi and Uncle Adam. You guys were dancing and playing kickball in the new playroom. You were so Healthy, Strong, Growing, meeting all your milestones then two weeks later you're gone. We knew right away what happened to you the day you passed away, there was nothing wrong with you. Healthy 20-month-olds don't just pass away. Mommy and I fought for you over and over every day while still in shock. We got connected with the right people sent your samples out, now we have proof of what we knew happened to you all along and we're going to change a lot of things. Those that are still sleeping and still don't believe better wake the f.. up before it happens to you. The truth is out and the proof is coming, this happened to the wrong family. Nobody is getting in my way. It's not about money for us. They can take their money and shove it up their ass. This should never have happened. All the money in the world would never stop me. They took you away from us and nothing can ever bring you back. My family is torn to pieces because of the poison in vaccines, now someone will pay. I promise we are going to change the world in your honor because of what happened to you. I won't stop until we do. Your now my little Angel guiding me everyday until we get justice for you and make changes before more children and families are destroyed. **#flyhighnicholas**🕊️🤍 we will do this together as long as we have to. One Starfish at a time. I'll never stop fighting for you. I love you Nicholas 💔🕊️🤍"

I am sure some of this anger and frustration is from dealing with government hoops, vaccine company immunity and the realization that one, or even hundreds, of parents who lost their child because of vaccine damage isn't going to easily change legislation on the matter.

Another Story:

Her Sweet Willow,

"Today is the same day that I took you to the doctor to get your 4 month shots. Before we left to go to the doctor I remember taking a picture of you in your green seat as you sat on the counter and watched me cook. It was a normal day. Your appointment was later in the afternoon. This would be the last picture that I would have of you normal.

Before we left to go to the doctor you were your normal self. Smiling so beautifully!

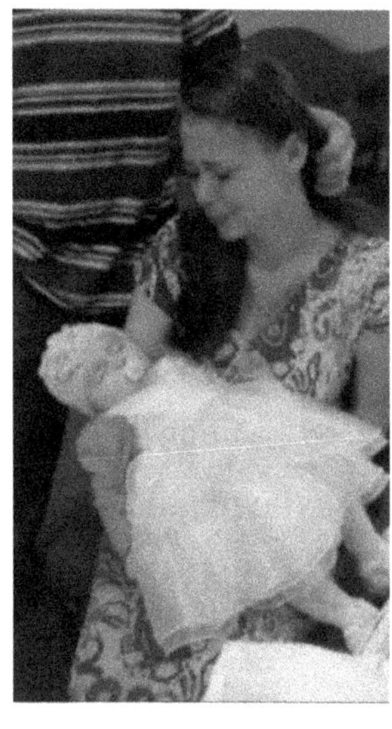

I didn't know that my decision I made this day to take you to the doctor would justify your fate. You were so happy as we left the house. I remember looking in the rear-view mirror and watching you play with your toys in your car seat as you smiled so sweetly! As we arrived to the doctor you were weighed. My heart felt happy when the nurse said you were 18 pounds! Growing so perfectly! We were sent back to the waiting room to wait for your name to be called. Moments later we were led to the back. I won't ever forget that room we were in asked to sit in as we waited for the doctor. Georgia Bulldog theme covered the walls. You continued to play with your toys as we waited for the doctor. The doctor arrived and he smiled as he looked at you! I won't ever forget him saying "Wow! Her smile just made my day because today has been a rough day"....as he nodded his head. I remember laughing and feeling so proud of you and the effect you had on others. You would always light any room you were in!

After the doctor assessed you ??and went over how healthy you were and how perfectly you were growing he left the room. The nurse arrived. As she arrived she had a tray with your vaccines . I undressed you and laid you on the table. She proceeded in doing what she came in there to do as she poked you the first time. You screamed, your face turned bloody red and she couldn't handle you as you fought her to stop. The nurse then asked me to hold you down for your final injections. This haunts me to this day. Your screams replay in my head. I did as I was asked thinking that what I was doing was to protect you! I held you down. You stared at me in agony. You had the Hep B, Prevnar 13, DTAP and rotavirus. The FDA approves 5mcg of aluminum as a safety measure , you were injected with almost 2,000 mcg of aluminum this day along with the aborted fetal cells, antifreeze, formaldehyde, ect...

As we left the doctor you screamed a high pitch scream for a matter of minutes in the backseat of the car and then fell asleep. This is when I lost you. When you awoke you were never the same, you were very lethargic. You were not yourself. You became very sickly instantly after. I tried to control your screams and your fevers. I thought I was doing the best that I could. You stopped eating and drinking .I kept telling myself you would get better! I was wrong, I had no idea that your soul was getting ready to leave mine. A few days later I found you. You were lifeless. Your brain hemorrhaged. You had a blood snot clot on your nose. I shook you and screamed for you to wake up and look at me. You never did...

You were gone. You were cold. I was so scared. Your heart had stopped beating as mine continued. The whole world stopped spinning. Your brain hemorrhaged from the heavy metals, your liver also. Your body was too weak for the overload of heavy metals and toxins. Everything was a blur ...I remember it felt like forever for a first responder to get there and it was only a matter of minutes. He didn't know you and I remember watching him from the porch as he tried so hard to bring you back, on the back of the bed of the truck, when I know in his heart that he knew you had been gone for awhile. I remember the cop stepped forward to walk up the steps of the porch and as he mumbled you were gone I screamed so loud nothing came out of my mouth, I was that scared. I remember having to make a decision so quickly rather to burn your body or bury you. Picking out your tiny dress and your coffin. I was given decisions that no mother should have to make. I miss you baby girl! Please stay with me the next few days because mommy is weak when it comes to you.

Since you have left, Mommy has fought. So have many others. We have traveled multiple times to the CDC in Atlanta, had many meetings at the Capital. Robert F Kennedy Jr also came to educate the legislators on the Bill HB416 that would teach parents the harm of vaccines and the tripled schedule & ingredients. Multiple billboards have been put up in your memory to educate others. Your story is worldwide along with thousands of other overwhelming stories that are the same as yours. You also have multiple songs that have been released in your honor. Your memory is definitely alive and you have saved so many! I'm so proud of you baby girl and the impact you have made from heaven! Your spirit is strong.

I'm so sorry for all of this baby, Mommy didn't know. I do promise you one thing your death will not be in vain! I won't allow it! You had a purpose and I'm watching it prevail.

Only one thing changed when you left.. "Everything."
#WeepForWillow

Shared with permission

My heart aches for this mom. She was a nurse and was one of those standing by that held her daughter down. No one in medical school or any hospital she ever worked at told her about the dangers of vaccines. She, like so many, suffered untold misery because of the protection of assets over the protection of innocent children. Stories like this can NOT be erased from our memory and history, though it is truly heart wrenching!

Another Story:
Chris Runquist, a mom whose twin daughters were severely damaged by Vaccines tells her story and I will put it here, in her own words:

"This is why I won't shut up about the damned vaccines!

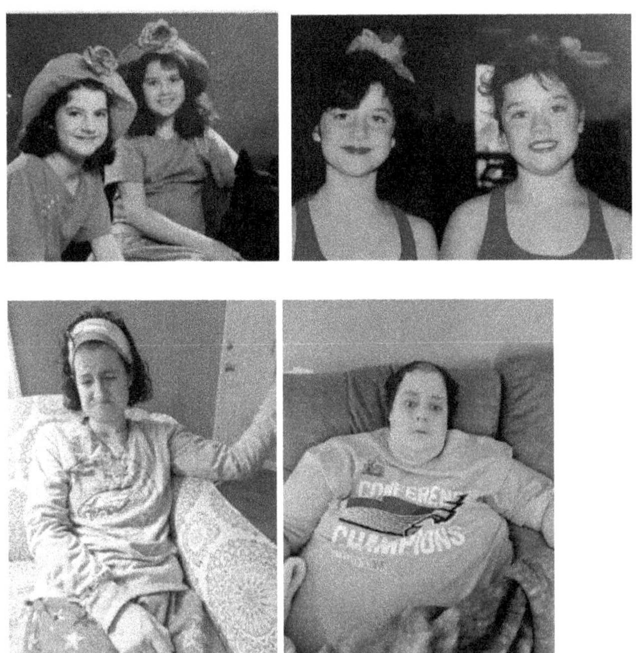

These are my twin daughters Jessica and Ashley. They were born normally, a month early for twins, in 1985. Except for medical hernia issues that Jessica had since infancy, they were happy and bright! You can see it in their eyes. They were in normal school and had lots of friends and lots of activities! Our dreams for them were optimistic and beautiful.

But then something happened in 1998, when they were 12 years old. They had the Hepatitis B shot for school. 20 minutes later, it was followed by anaphylaxis, blue lips, projectile vomiting, and seizure-like flailing of the arms and eyes rolling back. The doctor yelled at me on the phone when I called her and insisted that it was not from the injections that she administered 20 minutes prior at the office.

Jessica's life was immediately set back and changed after this. She never ever functioned at her full potential ever again after that shot. She was finally diagnosed with Autism in her teenage years. Complex medical issues followed her throughout her life.

Ashley, on the other hand recovered from this episode, after a week or so, but did go on to have occasional blackouts and would fall unconscious. The doctors called it Syncope, and one of her spinal tests confirmed that it could be Guillian Barre Syndrome. Ashley continued to work very hard through all of this. She was even on the Dean's List in college but continued to have the blackouts. In 2008 Ashley ended up in the hospital needing blood transfusions and her life went downhill fast after that. She was eventually diagnosed with Early Onset Alzheimer's.

Today, both Ashley and Jessica are totally disabled, have extreme difficulty with communication, wear diapers and are incontinent and need 24/7 care. That spark in their eyes faded a long time ago, and so did our dreams for their future."

This post was shared on Facebook, complete with pictures of their beautiful girls: smiling, happy and beautiful. Perfect, and then pictures of them in their current condition. Truly Heartbreaking.

On its original share date, it was also accompanied by over 860 comments, many of whom were sharing their own personal testimonies and histories of vaccine damage or damage done to a loved one. I wish you could read all the comments for yourself: from babies a few months old to kids in their teens. An 18 mo. old, loses eye contact and personality, a healthy, thriving 4 year old, turned to a vegetable, and now requires diapering at 16 years old. Another mom tells how she took hundreds of photos before age one, showing a healthy thriving little girl who, after the MMR, stopped looking at her mother, smiling and playing with her brother. A student in medical school suffers auto-immune issues after having to take the Hep. B for medical school. Children turned autistic, lost control of their bowels, were unable to speak or communicate, no longer able to run and play, no longer able to dress or feed themselves. Not only are their lives forever changed, but so are their parents'. From devastation and dashed hopes and dreams to fighting for survival. This damage impacts whole families and communities and typically lasts their whole lives.

This is not fake. None of these people have any reason to make any of their stories up. It earns them nothing, and for many of them it causes them to lose even more simply by speaking up. I know the stories are in the millions, at the very least, and yet this book will only hold a small fraction of them.

Here's a more recent story:

Healthy Infant Dies 13 Days After 2 Month Vaccines: Baby Vincent's Story

June 24, 2024

"On November 2, 2023, two-month-old baby Vincent Schambach was brought to his pediatrician for the routine two month well baby visit, where he received the following four vaccines, one of them a 5-in-1 combination shot:

Vincent was found unresponsive 13 days after the 2 month vaccines. Autopsy found cerebral and pulmonary edema along with spinal cord and liver congestion.
Vincent Schambach
8/29/2023 - 11/15/2023
circleofmamas.com for more information

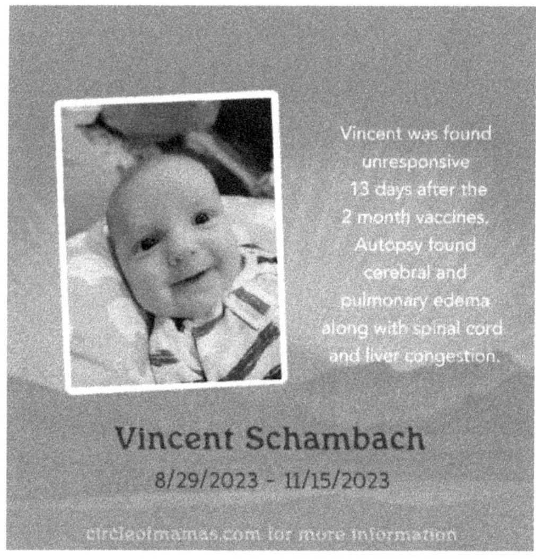

- Hib vaccine (Pedvax HIB by Merck Sharp & Dohme)
- Rotavirus Vaccine (RotaTeq by Merck Sharp & Dohme)
- DTaP-HepB-IPV (Pediarix by GlaxoSmithKline)
- Pneumococcal Conjugate 20-Valent (Prevnar 20 by Pfizer)

Over the next several days, Vincent had some vaccine side effects such as a low fever and an unusual choking cough– the doctors said it was all normal. Just 13 days after the vaccinations, Vincent was found unresponsive and was not able to be revived. Here is Vincent's story in his mother's own words:

"Vincent Schambach was born 8/29/2023 and passed in his sleep 11/15/2023, 13 days after his 2 month old vaccinations.

He was a strong, healthy, happy and super loved boy up until the week of his vaccinations. Immediately following his 2 month old shots, Vincent developed a 100 degree fever along with a cough that sounded like he was choking and gagging that would also turn his face bright red.

The doctors advised us to just keep giving him Tylenol and make sure he keeps drinking and having wet diapers which he did. The symptoms lasted for 4 days.

A week later, baby Vincent was found unresponsive in the morning along with frothy, blood-tinged, bubbly liquid coming out of his nose. Just when we thought the worst was over, he died and we have been devastated ever since.

The signs can be so subtle to the point you don't realize something is seriously wrong and a baby has no voice to tell us. We received the autopsy report 6 months later with a diagnosis of cerebral and pulmonary edema along with spinal cord and liver congestion.

The Dtap vaccine which Vincent received during his 2 month visit is known for a side effect of encephalitis (cerebral edema) which we are now trying to fight in court.

*Thoughts, prayers and justice for our sweet Vincent* 💔🙏

Shared from his mother, Lauren Seeger."

## The Numbers are Many

It was about 7 years ago when I watched the "VAXXED" documentary with many stories just as heart breaking as those I just shared. On the "VAXXED bus" there are over 4,000 names of vaccine injured or dead individuals. Their stories are gut wrenching and devastating. (If you'd like to watch the series, please see the links to all three documentaries in the Appendix sect.) While I do feel the need to go into the science of why and how, this is not just possible but probable and inescapable: that the ingredients in vaccines as well as the method they are administered should cause damage, but, truly, the greatest "proof" is in stories just like this.

Noteworthy, is the fact that at the end of the snippet of the story on Facebook about the triplets are links to over 30 peer reviewed articles from the National Library of Medicine that show how ingredients in vaccines can and do cause autism. There is also a great deal of information and other stories on these informational websites. (Please check out some of these sites listed in the Appendix for yourself)

While the injected virus does (or at least can) alter DNA pathways, even more deadly are the adjuvants, like Aluminum, Mercury and Thimerosal. These ingredients overwhelm the immune system and detoxification processes, can cross the "blood-brain barrier," causing neurological and neurodevelopmental problems, and compromise physiological systems and the autonomic nervous system. Vaccines injected directly into the bloodstream, bypasses all normal cellular responses and detox pathways, such as lymphatic and other excretory systems. (We will discuss this more in subsequent chapters.)

The National Institutes of Health admit that autism rates have climbed substantially. “Prior to the 1930’s and the introduction of vaccines, autism was virtually unknown.” It has also been stated that, “by 2006 the occurrence of autism had reached pandemic proportions.” From 3-5 in 10,000 to 1 in 166. The increase in number of vaccines has most certainly played a role in this, and an honest look at even the limited studies on the matter, prove this.

Autism is not the only health issue caused by vaccines (or at the very least vaccine influenced). Mild “flu like symptoms”, numbness and tingling, headaches, infertility, “brain fog”, paralysis, auto-immune diseases, allergies, inflammation of all kinds, organ damage, sudden onset diabetes, liver failure, nerve pain -the list is practically endless- and of course, death, are all possible consequences of vaccine damage.

The real pandemic, I believe, is that despite the repeated and horrific dangers and devastation caused by vaccination, people still believe in it. They still uphold and cling to it. They still believe that, despite the horrors, there is something to be gained by it. Even the most distinguished and accused “anti-vaxer” claims, repeatedly, "I'm not Anti-vaccine. I'm pro-vaccine. I'm just pro-choice, or Pro-science or pro-safety." Even our acclaimed and proactive Bobby Kennedy has stated, over and over again, that he is not anti-vaccine. Why Not?? Why will no one stand up against this atrocity of evil and proclaim the TRUTH, the REAL TRUTH: that vaccines NEVER DID and NEVER WILL have anything advantageous to offer us?? I am going to say this again later, because it bears repeating, but we are far from done. We have a lot more to talk about and have barely begun to state the case against vaccines.

# CHAPTER 4

## VACCINES AND THEIR INGREDIENTS

### DTAP

Here is a vaccine that is rushed to be administered anytime you get a cut, especially, God forbid, the proverbial “rusty nail.” The Tetanus, or more appropriately called, DTap is a vaccine I have gotten and given to my own children, before realizing how unnecessary it truly is! (We discover more why later in chapter 7)

This story on the tetanus shot - Shared from a fellow mom (who will remain anonymous) On June 22, 2023, demonstrates some of the mis-information and lack of knowledge that generally accompanies the administration of this injection. First of all, the tetanus shot is not administered alone, it is included in the DTaP - Diphtheria, Tetanus and Pertussis.

Story from a mom who took her child to the emergency room with a cut:

Doctor: "We're going to give her a tetanus vaccine."

Mom: "Really? What brand and configuration did you have in mind?"

Doctor: "Just Tetanus."

Mom: "You mean the DTaP?"

Doctor: "Well, yes."

Mom: "So, you want to give my child a vaccine for 3 diseases when you're only concerned about one?"

Doctor: "It's the only way it comes." (wrong)

Mom: "So...how long will it take for the vaccine to help her create antibodies against tetanus?"

Doctor: "About 3 weeks."

Mom: "If this wound contains tetanus spores in the correct environment, how long before the spores start producing toxins causing lockjaw then death?"

Doctor: "Immediately."

Mom: "So you want to give her a vaccine that she won't mount an immune response with until about a week after she's dead, then?"

We left without the shot or TiG...

Scares me that I have more information than a physician.

It should scare you, too."

Fun facts on tetanus that clearly most doctors don't know (or lie about) since they give the DTaP vaccine for even sinus infections and any minor cut:

1. Tetanus is an anaerobic bacteria, meaning it can't survive in oxygenated environments meaning if the wound bled, NO tetanus.

2. Just because you get cut on metal (rusty or not), it doesn't automatically mean tetanus bacteria is present. Tetanus (C. Tetani) is normally found in manure/dirt and not on a clean plumbing fixture.

3. Even if there was a deep puncture wound that did not bleed, caused by an object that had tetanus bacteria on it, you literally can NOT "vaccinate" against a bacterial infection AFTER the exposure. The vaccine is not an instant tetanus killer; it would take weeks for your body to produce enough antibodies (provided the vaccine is even successful at all).

4. If there were serious concerns about tetanus exposure (as previously explained) then the ONLY thing that could help (outside of allowing the wound to bleed, if possible, and cleaning the wound with soap, water, or hydrogen peroxide) would be the TiG shot (tetanus immunoglobulin), which is an anti-toxin and not a vaccine.

5. There is no "tetanus vaccine" available in the United States, only the DTaP which is a 3-in-1 cocktail vaccine consisting of Diphtheria, Tetanus & Pertussis (whooping cough) or Td (tetanus and diphtheria).

To summarize:

1. A tetanus shot would not help a current case of tetanus as a vaccine takes several weeks to create antibodies. If a current case of tetanus is truly a concern, the TiG shot is what should be

given.

2. According to the VAERS database, reactions to vaccines for tetanus and diphtheria are not rare. As of August 2012, there were over 22,000 adverse reactions reported and 67 deaths.

3. Lastly, the CDC states that efficacy of the tetanus toxoid has never been studied in a vaccine trial."

May I point out, here that deaths in the US from Tetanus are so rare there are no records for it (It is essentially Zero). I truly appreciate this woman's candor and wisdom on the subject. I would only add that I don't think the TiG shot should be considered either (we will talk more about anti-toxins and Immune Globulins later in this chapter).

I want to include a few snippets from a documentary on the DTap, from 1982, then called DPT, to give us some historical context before we move on to more recent data, called, "DPT: Vaccine roulette" Produced by Lea Thompson from WRC -tv in Washington by The National Vaccine Information Center.
The part of the vaccine, then, most being considered was the Pertussis, or Whooping Cough Vaccine.

It was required of school age children to receive 4 doses of the DPT before they were allowed to go to school. These vaccines were promoted as part of a health regime, yet as was pointed out in the video, they were shown to cause "damage to a devastating degree."

Doctor Mendelsohn, a pediatrician and author, is quoted as saying that the DPT is “probably the poorest and most dangerous of all the vaccines.” Also, that it is the “most unstable and least reliable vaccine we give our children.”

At the same time, a Dr. Edward Mortimer, with his many degrees, and part of the Academy of Pediatrics, proclaims, loudly, “The benefits of the vaccine, in my view, far outweigh the risks!”

Dr. Gordan Stewart, a British Epidemiologist (one who observes and studies the outcomes of disease), proclaims, “I believe that the risk of damage from the vaccine is now greater than the risk of damage from disease.”

Still, Dr. John Robbins from the FDA (and no surprise), unwaveringly declares, that, “despite its complications, whooping cough vaccine... is something that should be given to children.”

Since 1933, it has been known that DTP causes brain damage.

The Pediatric Red Book from 1977, lists the severe reactions to DTP as

High Fever

Collapse

Shock-like collapse

Unconsolable crying

Convulsions

Brain Damage

It is even correlated to SIDS (sudden infant death syndrome)

The documentary, found on Bit chute, is nearly an hour long, but could be helpful for those who want to be further educated about the history of the risks and damage of one of the most prescribed vaccines in our nation's history. Although, the rates of damage are, I believe, grossly underrated, as they have been throughout vaccine history.

It is sad, indeed, that this cycle and the stories of the lives impacted and forever damaged must continue. It is also disturbing to watch those with vested interests continue to defend and be the instruments used to continue the devastating epidemic of vaccine use and the mutilation caused by it. This, indeed, is where love of money, prestige and position become very dark and evil. Where they trump love of mankind and the good of others and future generations.

Another story:

September 22, 2021

(I'm keeping the story and comments as I originally found them.)

One DTaP Shot Paralyzed Baby Nash from the Neck Down

"It's truly unbelievable what is happening to perfectly healthy babies, and people just don't get it.

- They don't get that vaccine injuries like this *aren't rare at all*.

- They don't get that the diseases we are vaccinating against aren't even posing an imminent danger to infants and children.
- That we are subjecting our children to a risk-filled procedure, for *no emergent reason*.
- They don't get that you could be **fully vaccinated**, *and still get that exact infection*.
- They don't get that a single vaccine injection could cause a *huge range* of vaccine injuries, including death, which are near impossible to predict.
- They don't get that you could be trading a short term or even asymptomatic infection that has treatments, for a potentially lifelong chronic illness which are inherently untreatable, which require dependency on pharmaceuticals for life.
- They don't get or they don't know that unvaccinated children are healthier than vaccinated children.
- They don't get that IF something does happen to your child, that *no one will believe you*, your medical providers may deny the vaccine was involved, and they may not be able to recover and help your child.
- They don't get that IF something happens, that there is no one who takes responsibility, that you can't hold the pharmaceutical company accountable, nor the government's no-fault system.

- They don't get that IF something happens, your medical provider may not report this reaction to VAERS, and without this important data collecting, statistically it's like it didn't happen. But as the parent, you know it did. And now you have to live the rest of your life knowing you were deceived, betrayed and gaslighted.

And this is how vaccines continue to be *believed* as "Safe and Effective" because no one *wants* to report reactions for vaccines, because it may create vaccine hesitancy, yet because of this overt refusal to acknowledge, report and study vaccine risks and harms–vaccine hesitancy is not only warranted, it's completely justified.

Baby Nash

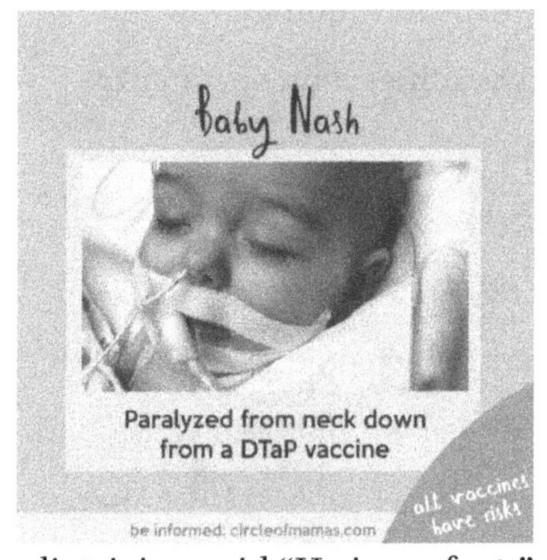


Baby Nash was born perfectly healthy. He was happy, beautiful, and growing perfectly and hitting every milestone on time. At his 6 month well-child checkup on January 22, 2021, his pediatrician said "He is perfect."

Baby Nash got one vaccine (cocktail) that day, just a single DTaP injection. His mother documented the days after the vaccine. (see link in Appendix)

The video shows footage of a healthy, thriving, bouncing baby for 12 days, and pictures of the 13th day, when he received the DTap. He is hospitalized with tubes down his throat, and clearly miserable while his mother tries to comfort him.

Feb 4th 2021 he was "life flighted" to Children's Hospital, where he would spend the next 2 months. The video ends declaring that "he wasn't even sick," and that she "isn't going down without a fight."

Unfortunately, I do not know how this story ends. Likely, this mom, or the parents, are still trying to fight through the court system, or perhaps even for their child's life.

Sadly, this story is mirrored by so many others just like it.

## INGREDIENTS

Some of the story is told through the ingredients alone. Ingredients that are bound (maybe almost guaranteed) to cause problems.

There are various trade names of the DTap and for clarity, I will name a few:

Adacel, Daptacel, Infanrix, Pediarix, Vaxelis and Boostrix. The Inserts are all similar. I am using information from the Daptacel brand insert here.

"DESCRIPTION [the numbers are contained in the insert under each new line. This was how far down I had to scroll to find any actual ingredients]

289 DAPTACEL is a sterile isotonic suspension of pertussis antigens and diphtheria and tetanus

290 toxoids adsorbed on aluminum phosphate, for intramuscular injection.

291 Each 0.5 mL dose contains 15 Lf diphtheria toxoid, 5 Lf tetanus toxoid and acellular pertussis

292 antigens [10 mcg detoxified pertussis toxin (PT), 5 mcg filamentous hemagglutinin (FHA), 3 mcg

293 pertactin (PRN), and 5 mcg fimbriae types 2 and 3 (FIM)].

294 Other ingredients per 0.5 mL dose include 1.5 mg aluminum phosphate (0.33 mg of aluminum) as 295 the adjuvant, ≤5 mcg residual formaldehyde, residual aldehydes are removed by ultrafiltration. The individual antigens are adsorbed separately

304 onto aluminum phosphate.

305 Corynebacterium diphtheriae is grown in modified Mueller's growth medium. (3) After

306 purification by ammonium sulfate fractionation, diphtheria toxin is detoxified with formaldehyde

307 and diafiltered. Clostridium tetani is grown in modified Mueller-Miller casamino acid medium

308 without beef heart infusion. (4) Tetanus toxin is detoxified with formaldehyde and purified by

309 ammonium sulfate fractionation and diafiltration. Diphtheria and tetanus toxoids are individually
310 adsorbed onto aluminum phosphate.
311 The adsorbed diphtheria, tetanus and acellular pertussis components are combined with aluminum
312 phosphate (as adjuvant), 2-phenoxyethanol (not as a preservative) and water for injection. Both diphtheria and tetanus toxoids induce at least 2 units of antitoxin per mL in the guinea pig
314 potency test. The potency of the acellular pertussis vaccine components is determined by the
315 antibody response of immunized mice to detoxified PT, FHA, PRN and FIM as measured by
316 enzyme-linked immunosorbent assay (ELISA).

The following adverse events have been spontaneously reported during the post-marketing use of
234 DAPTACEL in the US and other countries. Because these events are reported voluntarily from a
235 population of uncertain size, it may not be possible to reliably estimate their frequency or
236 establish a causal relationship to vaccine exposure.
237 The following adverse events were included based on one or more of the following factors:
238 severity, frequency of reporting, or strength of evidence for a causal relationship to DAPTACEL.

• Blood and lymphatic disorders

240 Lymphadenopathy

241 • Cardiac disorders

242 Cyanosis

243 • Gastro-intestinal disorders  Nausea, diarrhea

245 • General disorders and administration site conditions

246 Local reactions: injection site pain, injection site rash, injection site nodule, injection site

247 mass, extensive swelling of injected limb (including swelling that involves adjacent joints).

248 • Infections and infestations

249 Injection site cellulitis, cellulitis, injection site abscess

250 • Immune system disorders

251 Hypersensitivity, allergic reaction, anaphylactic reaction (edema, face edema, swelling face,

252 pruritus, rash generalized) and other types of rash (erythematous, macular, maculo-papular)

253 • Nervous system disorders

254 Convulsions: febrile convulsion, grand mal convulsion, partial seizures

255 HHE, hypotonia, somnolence, syncope

256 • Psychiatric disorders

257 Screaming”

## Some snippets of a study by EBioMedicine on DTP

"abstract Article history: Received 4, June 2016, Received in revised form 21 January 2017 Accepted 29 January 2017 Available online 1, February 2017, Background: We examined the introduction of diphtheria-tetanus-pertussis (DTP) and oral polio vaccine (OPV) in an urban community in Guinea-Bissau in the early 1980s.

Methods: The child population had been followed with 3-monthly nutritional weighing sessions since 1978. From June 1981 DTP and OPV were offered from 3 months of age at these sessions. Due to the 3-monthly intervals between sessions, the children were allocated by birthday in a 'natural experiment' to receive vaccinations early or late between 3 and 5 months of age. We included children who were 6 months of age when vaccinations started and children born until the end of December 1983. We compared mortality between 3 and 5 months of age of DTP-vaccinated and not-yet-DTP-vaccinated children in Cox proportional hazard models. Results: Among 3–5-month-old children, having received DTP (±OPV) was associated with a mortality hazard ratio (HR) of 5.00 (95% CI 1.53–16.3) compared with not-yet-DTP-vaccinated children. Differences in background factors did not explain the effect. The negative effect was particularly strong for children who had received DTP only and no OPV (HR = 10.0 (2.61–38.6)).

All-cause infant mortality after 3 months of age increased after the introduction of these vaccines (HR = 2.12 (1.07–4.19)).

Conclusion: DTP was associated with increased mortality; OPV may modify the effect of DTP. 

"The Introduction of Diphtheria-Tetanus-Pertussis and Oral Polio Vaccine Among Young Infants in an Urban African Community: A Natural Experiment

Søren Wengel Mogensen a,1 , Andreas Andersen b,1 , Amabelia Rodrigues a , Christine S Benn b,c , Peter Aaby a

**Conclusions**

DTP was associated with 5-fold higher mortality than being unvaccinated. No prospective study has shown beneficial survival effects of DTP. Unfortunately, DTP is the most widely used vaccine, and the proportion who receives DTP3 is used globally as an indicator of the performance of national vaccination programs. It should be of concern that the effect of routine vaccinations on all-cause mortality was not tested in randomized trials. All currently available evidence suggests that DTP vaccine may kill more children from other causes than it saves from diphtheria, tetanus or pertussis. Though a vaccine protects children against the target disease it may simultaneously increase susceptibility to unrelated infections. The recently published SAGE review called for randomized trials of DTP (Higgins et al., 2014). However, at the same time the IVIR-AC committee to which SAGE delegated the follow-up studies of the NSEs of vaccines has indicated that it will not be possible to examine the effect of DTP in an unbiased way. If that decision by IVIR-AC remains unchallenged, the present study may remain the closest we will ever come to a RCT of the NSEs of DTP."

This admission, from a source that still upholds the efficacy of DTP vaccine is about the best and most honest of all the studies I can find, for they have been conducted by companies that favor vaccines and manufacturers and Never truly compare Vaccinated to unvaccinated individuals in true placebo-based trials.

I would also add that DTP indeed does NOT protect from the target disease, and there are no proofs to be found that it ever has. We will talk about this more in the "*Theory* and *Science*" sections.

For now, let's take a deeper look at the other vaccines.

## MMR

Another story shared by Nick Catone on Nov. 13th, 2017
By Mom: **Ariana Franklin**

"My son got the measles from his 12-month shots and ended up in the hospital for 3 days. I was never warned of the adverse reactions and definitely never told the MMR is a live vaccine so that I could keep my child away from babies and other people so he couldn't shed around them. Of course they're not going to tell you any of that since they get paid for it. My baby boy could have died in the hospital and it was definitely one of the most scariest times of my life. Thank God he came out OK and got to come home. I switched his doctors and I had a long talk with his new one which is for parents choice on vaccines and I told him I didn't want to do it anymore. So he told me what I needed to do to keep his immune system strong. So he gets a probiotic every morning and has a healthy diet. A year later, he will be two this month, he's in the 80th percentile and his doctor is amazed at how healthy he is. No issues at all and hasn't got sick once."

The picture shows a little boy, clearly covered in measles (though it may not be so clear in this print). What is profound about the story, which is certainly not an isolated story, is that you can and often do get measles from the MMR vaccine. It stands to logic and reason that this would certainly be possible. They are literally injecting you with the disease. Why would anyone think it impossible or unlikely that children will develop measles from a measles toxoid, or live virus? (For clarification, as we discuss this later, even if it is understood that a "virus" is not a living organism,

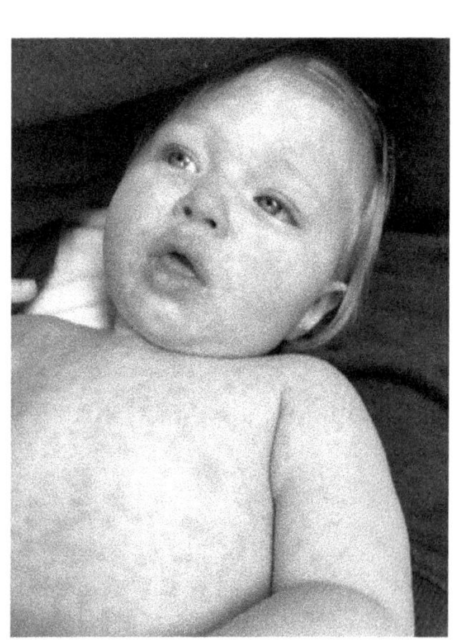

still, the components are surrounded by actively infectious microbes.)

## DESCRIPTION

## (from the vaccine insert)

"M-M-R® II (Measles, Mumps, and Rubella Virus Vaccine Live) is a live virus vaccine for vaccination against measles (rubeola), mumps, and rubella (German measles). M-M-R II is a sterile lyophilized preparation of

(1) ATTENUVAX® (Measles Virus Vaccine Live), a more attenuated line of measles virus, derived from Enders' attenuated Edmonston strain and propagated in chick embryo cell culture;

(2) MUMPSVAX® (Mumps Virus Vaccine Live), the Jeryl Lynn™ (B level) strain of mumps virus propagated in chick embryo cell culture; and

(3) MERUVAX® II (Rubella Virus Vaccine Live), the Wistar RA 27/3 strain of live attenuated rubella virus propagated in WI-38 human diploid lung fibroblasts.

{1,2} The growth medium for measles and mumps is Medium 199 (a buffered salt solution containing vitamins and amino acids and supplemented with fetal bovine serum) containing SPGA (sucrose, phosphate, glutamate, and recombinant human albumin) as stabilizer and neomycin. The growth medium for rubella is Minimum Essential Medium (MEM) [a buffered salt solution containing vitamins and amino acids and supplemented with fetal bovine serum] containing recombinant human albumin and neomycin. Sorbitol and hydrolyzed gelatin stabilizer are added to the individual virus harvests. The cells, virus pools, and fetal bovine serum are all screened for the absence of adventitious agents. The reconstituted vaccine is for subcutaneous administration. Each 0.5 mL dose contains not less than 1,000 TCID50 (tissue culture infectious doses) of measles virus; 12,500 TCID50 of mumps virus; and 1,000 TCID50 of rubella virus. Each dose of the vaccine is calculated to contain sorbitol (14.5 mg), sodium phosphate, sucrose (1.9 mg), sodium chloride, hydrolyzed gelatin (14.5 mg), recombinant human albumin (≤0.3 mg), fetal bovine serum

Note: There are many who question or wonder whether vaccines contain human tissue cells and/or fetal tissue cells. From the very inception of vaccine creation, they contain products derived from diseased human tissue: Human Diploid cells, such as those from lung tissue (see above), TCID50 (Cultured diseased tissue), recombinant human DNA (albumin) literally means the combining of two different organisms (or species) or DNA molecules. These are just a few examples. WI-38 and MRC-5 are cell lines from aborted fetal tissue used in the creation and culturing of vaccines including MMR.

## ADVERSE REACTIONS

"The following adverse reactions are listed in decreasing order of severity, without regard to causality, within each body system category and have been reported during clinical trials, with use of the marketed vaccine, or with use of monovalent or bivalent vaccine containing measles, mumps, or rubella:

Body as a Whole Panniculitis; atypical measles; fever; syncope; headache; dizziness; malaise; irritability. Cardiovascular System Vasculitis.

Digestive System Pancreatitis; diarrhea; vomiting; parotitis; nausea.

Endocrine System Diabetes mellitus.

Hemic and Lymphatic System Thrombocytopenia (see WARNINGS, Thrombocytopenia); purpura; regional lymphadenopathy; leukocytosis.

Immune System Anaphylaxis and anaphylactoid reactions have been reported as well as related phenomena such as angioneurotic edema (including peripheral or facial edema) and bronchial spasm in individuals with or without an allergic history.

Musculoskeletal System Arthritis; arthralgia; myalgia. Arthralgia and/or arthritis (usually transient and rarely chronic), and polyneuritis are features of infection with wild-type rubella and vary in frequency and severity with age and sex, being greatest in adult females and least in prepubertal children. This type of involvement as well as myalgia and paresthesia, have also been reported following the administration of MERUVAX II. Chronic arthritis has been associated with wild-type rubella infection and has been related to persistent virus and/or viral antigen isolated from body tissues. Only rarely have vaccine recipients developed chronic joint symptoms. Following vaccination in children, reactions in joints are uncommon and generally of brief duration. In women, incidence rates for arthritis and arthralgia are generally higher than those seen in children (children: 0-3%; women: 12-26%),{17,56,57} and the reactions tend to be more marked and of longer duration. Symptoms may persist for a matter of months or on rare occasions for years. In adolescent girls, the reactions appear to be intermediate in incidence between those seen in children and in adult women. Even in women older than 35 years, these reactions are generally well tolerated and rarely interfere with normal activities.

Nervous System Encephalitis; encephalopathy; measles inclusion body encephalitis (MIBE) (see CONTRAINDICATIONS); subacute sclerosing panencephalitis (SSPE); Guillain-Barré Syndrome (GBS); acute disseminated encephalomyelitis (ADEM); transverse myelitis; febrile convulsions; afebrile convulsions or seizures; ataxia; polyneuritis; polyneuropathy; ocular palsies; paresthesia. The risk of serious neurological disorders following live measles virus vaccine administration remains less than the risk of encephalitis and encephalopathy following infection with wild-type measles (1 per 1000 reported cases).{58,59} In severely immunocompromised individuals who have been inadvertently vaccinated with measles containing vaccine; measles inclusion body encephalitis, pneumonitis, and fatal outcome as a direct consequence of disseminated measles vaccine virus infection have been reported (see CONTRAINDICATIONS). In this population, disseminated mumps and rubella vaccine virus infection have also been reported. There have been reports of subacute sclerosing panencephalitis (SSPE) in children who did not have a history of infection with wild-type measles but did receive measles vaccine. Some of these cases may have resulted from unrecognized measles in the first year of life or possibly from the measles vaccination. Based on estimated nationwide measles vaccine distribution, the association of SSPE cases to measles vaccination is about one case per million vaccine doses distributed. This is far less than the association with infection with wild-type measles, 6-22 cases of SSPE per million cases of measles. The results of a retrospective case-controlled study conducted by the Centers for Disease Control and Prevention suggest that the overall effect of measles vaccine has been to protect against SSPE by preventing measles with its inherent higher risk of SSPE.{60} Cases of aseptic meningitis have been reported to VAERS following measles, mumps, and rubella vaccination. Although a causal relationship between the Urabe strain of mumps vaccine and aseptic meningitis has been shown, there is no evidence to link Jeryl Lynn™ mumps vaccine to aseptic meningitis.

Respiratory System Pneumonia: pneumonitis (see CONTRAINDICATIONS); sore throat; cough; rhinitis. Skin Stevens-Johnson syndrome; erythema multiforme; urticaria; rash; measles-like rash; pruritis. Local reactions including burning/stinging at injection site; wheal and flare; redness (erythema); swelling; induration; tenderness; vesiculation at injection site; Henoch-Schönlein purpura; acute hemorrhagic edema of infancy.

Special Senses — Ear Nerve deafness; otitis media. Special Senses — Eye Retinitis; optic neuritis; papillitis; retrobulbar neuritis; conjunctivitis.

Urogenital System Epididymitis; orchitis.

Other Death from various, and in some cases unknown, causes has been reported rarely following vaccination with measles, mumps, and rubella vaccines; however, a causal relationship has not been established in healthy individuals (see CONTRAINDICATIONS)."

While that was a slew of information and enormous number of adverse reactions they admit having been reported, I do not believe their highly conservative numbers, as it does not line up with the number of cases that have suffered violently from this vaccine. Nor do I believe any of their hype about "wild-type measles." We will talk more near the end of this chapter about where the data for the statistics they are referencing come from.

Also, it is certainly note-worthy that you can, indeed get measles from the vaccine (and not measles only), and there is other evidence that could prove that the vaccine, itself, is keeping this disease in circulation and contributing, if not causing the measles outbreaks of today.

The following is a transcript from Dr. Toni Bark while testifying at a House Xommittee in Washington.

## Measles On the Rise?

"February 28, 2019

My name is Dr. Toni Bark and I am a licensed MD in the state of Illinois. I am trained in pediatrics and rehabilitative medicine and I directed a pediatric emergency room in the inner city of Chicago. During that time, I witnessed several children, after being in the vaccine clinic, presenting to the emergency room in status epilepticus, with asthma and even respiratory arrest. That was a while ago.

Since that time, there has been an emerging field called epigenetics. Epigenetics is the field of looking at the link between genetics and environmental toxins affecting people individually. Vaccines are not safe and effective for everyone. They cannot be one size fits all. [No other medical procedure is mandated for everyone regardless of risk.] Not everyone has the same risk factors. In the last 20-30 years we have elucidated some things that are known as risk factors, and they are called Single Nucleotide Polymorphic Variants. These interface with things like drugs and vaccines very differently for different people. Serious adverse reactions to vaccination are not a one-in-a-million event. There can be maybe up to 10-15% of people who are quite susceptible to different vaccines. This is a [sizable] minority, a susceptible minority, who are being left out in the rain without an umbrella. So, while it sounds good and well that vaccines are safe and effective, just so you understand, they are legally classified as unavoidably unsafe, and the manufacturers are not liable.

This is a liability-free product that is being mandated on children who may have epigenetic susceptibility to injury from these liability-free products. The injuries are serious and include death and chronic encephalopathies as well as chronic autoimmunity. While there have only been two deaths from measles in this country since 2003, there have been at least 450 [or so] children who have died from the vaccine. [And, since CDC's own Harvard Pilgrim HMO study of the Vaccine Adverse Event Reporting System showed less than 1% of vaccine adverse events are ever reported, the death rate is likely many times greater.]

Gregory Poland, a vaccinologist at Mayo Clinic, has written an article that cites *The Paradox of Measles* which states that you "cannot eradicate a virus like measles with a live viral vaccine" (due to shedding of live virus and failure of the vaccine). You also will see that the majority of outbreaks of measles cases around the country are actually in the vaccinated. So, this is a complex picture, it is not one-sided, there are a lot of grey areas; this is a complex issue. The [other side] would have you believe that it is not complex, that vaccines are safe and effective, that the vaccine prevents measles, and that if everyone was vaccinated there would not be measles and that is not true. The largest outbreak New York City has seen in recent years was just a few years ago (2011) and it was started by a 22-year-old recent recipient of an MMR booster. And 35-40 people who had all been vaccinated got a vaccine strain measles.

In Corpus Christi 1983 there were over 400 students who had all been vaccinated, 98% vaccination rates, 97% of which had antibodies, memory antibodies and they still got measles. There are dozens of examples of outbreaks in highly (97% and above) vaccinated populations. This is not a clear black-and-white picture. And, while the Disney outbreak was assumed to be due to the unvaccinated, this is far from the reality. During the 2015 California measles outbreak, many suspected cases occurred in persons who were recently vaccinated. One-hundred-ninety-four (194) measles virus sequences were collected in 2015, with 73 cases found to have actually been vaccine-strain measles. (Roy F, Mendoza L, Hiebert J et al. Rapid Identification of Measles Virus Vaccine Genotype by Real-Time PCR. J Clin Microbiol. 2017 Mar;55(3):735-743).

The CDC-recommended requirements for medical exemption are lagging about 30 years behind the science of the epigenetic risk factors entering medical exemptions far and few. In addition, most doctors are fearful of writing such exemptions as they worry they will be labeled “anti-vaxxers” and possibly brought before their state’s ethics committee. If you eliminate the exemptions you are making a large minority of people susceptible to very serious risks including death. You are also going to see many students opting for homeschooling until that becomes illegal. You are also creating a mood of extreme distrust of government. I consult with patients all over the country, as a specialist treating vaccine-related injuries including seizures, and GI disorders. I have also testified as an expert witness for injured families in the VICP. The Federal Table of Injuries for the MMR includes injuries such as encephalitis, chronic encephalopathy, chronic arthritis, measles, chronic thrombocytopenic purpura, and more. In addition, over 450 deaths have been reported to VAERS due to the vaccine but with less than 1% of adverse events being reported and in light of the manufacturer itself deciding if deaths are related to the vaccine, it is doubtful this number reflects the actual number of deaths from the vaccine.

I oppose any bill that mandates medical procedures, which come with risks, immunizes the manufacturer of liability, and violates informed consent/international law on informed consent. As a physician, I took an oath to do what is best for my individual patients and to first do no harm. I don't plan on acting against my oath. Thank you

Toni Bark MD MHEM LEED AP

## What is Measles, Mumps and Rubella?

According to the Mayo Clinic, **MUMPS** is an illness caused by a virus that affects the glands on each side of the face which can become swollen, tender or painful, and is, supposedly, highly contagious. They claim there is no specific medicine or treatment for mumps, only treatment for pain & discomfort.

Although they claim mumps is a disease no one gets any more due to vaccines, I have certainly noted the same exact symptoms (or detox reactions) in myself and others before. It appears that mumps is not a "threat" in the US anymore and no one ever talks about it, and I have not heard of a "case of mumps" in my whole life. (We will address some of these disease symptoms in a later chapter, but for now we will not focus on mumps.)

**Rubella**, which is also known as German measles, is, supposedly, a viral infection that causes a mild rash and other symptoms. It's gravest concern is for birth defects in pregnant women who have rubella. It is even stated that one could get rubella and not even notice. Makes me wonder if anyone actually has a definitive definition or diagnosis for Rubella, and I'm inclined to believe that it would more likely be pulled from a diagnosis book when needed, to blame something on or find an excuse for.

For this book, we are just going to focus on measles which, for now, is the number one reason why people are vaccinated with MMR.

## So, **what is** Measles?

You can easily find info on what is commonly believed about measles on the internet. I am going to quote from information on the Circle of Mammas Website (much of the articles used are from The National Library of Medicine):

"Measles is a viral respiratory illness characterized by runny nose, fever, conjunctivitis, cough, and by a flat, red spotted rash." So, really, the thing that makes it stand out from other detox sicknesses is the rash, and the severity.

"Prior to the introduction of the very first measles vaccine in 1963, nearly all children had measles by the time they reached 15 years old. While many infectious diseases in eras past had notoriously high mortality rates, this was largely due to poverty, malnutrition and overcrowding–factors which increase the overall vulnerability of a person to a range of diseases.

By the 1950s and 1960s, the living conditions and nutritional status of children had improved to the degree that measles became a mild, but obligatory, part of childhood–like chickenpox in the 80's. Even the 1960's TV show *The Brady Bunch* time-capsuled the prevailing attitude at the time about measles in an entire episode where all six kids 'got the measles.'

Infections with measles virus range from completely asymptomatic, to mild, to more severe, including fatal–the predictors of severe outcomes often have to do with host susceptibility and conditions (nutritional status / vitamin A deficiency, overall health, underlying conditions, HIV status, etc). Severe measles outcomes are typically rare in a healthy, well-nourished child who doesn't have a serious underlying medical condition."

"Measles Severity / Complications

**Vitamin A deficiency** is associated with severe measles-related complications in children and adults, delaying recovery and promoting xerophthalmia, corneal ulcer, and blindness. Acute measles precipitates vitamin A deficiency by depleting vitamin A stores and increasing its utilization, leading to more severe ocular injury. Vitamin A supplementation given to children with measles has been associated with reduced severe disease and death rates.

A **1992 study** examined the vitamin A levels of 89 children younger than 2 years old with measles in New York and they found that vitamin A levels decrease during measles even in children who were not deficient, and that children with low levels of vitamin A were more likely to have high fever, have a fever for 7 days or more, and more likely to be hospitalized. Children with low vitamin A also had lower measles-specific antibody levels.

I am guessing that lower nutrition in itself is a defining factor of measles complications.

<u>Common to rare measles complications</u>

- **Diarrhea and vomiting.** (8% of cases) Diarrhea and vomiting can result in losing too much water from the body (dehydration).
- **Ear infection.** (7% – 9% of cases)

- **Bronchitis, laryngitis or croup.** Measles may lead to irritation and swelling (inflammation) of the airways (croup). It can also lead to inflammation of the inner walls that line the main air passageways of the lungs (bronchitis). Measles can also cause inflammation of the voice box (laryngitis).
- **Pneumonia.** (1% – 6% of cases) An infection of the lungs.
- **Encephalitis.** (1 in 1,000-2,000 persons) Encephalitis is irritation and swelling (inflammation) of the brain. More common in people with weakened immune systems or other underlying conditions. Typically manifests with a triad of symptoms comprising fever, headache and altered level of consciousness.
- **Subacute sclerosing panencephalitis (SSPE)** is a rare (1 per 100,000 cases) and fatal degenerative central nervous system disease caused by a persistent infection with a mutant measles virus. The onset is several years after the episode of measles (on average seven years) and most affected children had measles before two years of age.
- **Pregnancy problems.** If you're pregnant and get measles, some complications could include premature birth, low birth weight and fetal demise. This is one reason why nature intended us to get measles in childhood.

According to this study, The Resurgence of Measles in the United States, 1989-1990, a total of 18,193 measles cases were reported in 1989 (of which 37% were vaccinated), and in 1990 a total of 27,786 cases were reported (of which 19% were vaccinated).

*"The measles epidemic of 1989-1990 was due primarily to widespread transmission of virus, particularly among unvaccinated preschool-aged children of racial and ethnic minority groups living in inner-city areas.[They say]*

*In this age group, the incidence of measles among blacks in 1989 and 1990 was 142 and 87 per 100,000, respectively, and among Hispanics it was 121 and 164 per 100,000, respectively, compared to 16 and 23 per 100,000 among non-Hispanic whites.*

A provisional total of 41 measles-associated deaths were reported in 1989 and 89 deaths reported in 1990; eight percent had been vaccinated; 60% of all deaths were under 5 years and 28% were over 20 years of age. Twelve percent of deaths had a serious underlying illness, including seven who were infected with HIV.

**Comment:** The case fatality rate for this 1989-1990 measles epidemic is higher than expected or observed in the period before the vaccine was introduced. Several factors could be influencing the higher case fatality rate: total cases were underreported (in fact many surveys from this period indicate that around 29% of cases were ever reported); the shift in cases to children under 5 and over 20 (when historically measles was more common in school-aged children); inappropriate medical care (were hospitalized cases given vitamin A?).

Great sources of Vit. A include:

- **Cod liver oil**
- **liver, fish**
- **Eggs**
- **Milk products**
- Orange and yellow-colored **vegetables** and **fruits.**
- Other sources of beta-carotene such as **broccoli**, **spinach**, and **most dark green, leafy vegetables**

According to the CDC website, the total cases of measles was 285 last year. There are no reported deaths in this number. They claim that measles was eradicated in 2000 and that only people coming into the US are spreading it. There is much more substantial evidence and science to support the fact that the cases and epidemics popping up are from vaccinated individuals.

For healthy individuals who have access to nutrition and cleanliness, measles is not a life-threatening condition or one that causes permanent damage. On the other hand, complications from the vaccination, itself are much more severe.

**From the package insert:**

- Panniculitis;
- atypical measles;
- fever; syncope;

- headache;
- dizziness;
- malaise;
- irritability.
- Digestive System Pancreatitis;
- diarrhea;
- vomiting;
- parotitis;
- nausea.
- Hematologic and Lymphatic Systems Thrombocytopenia;
- purpura;
- regional lymphadenopathy;
- leukocytosis.
- Immune System Anaphylaxis,
- anaphylactoid reactions,
- angioedema (including peripheral or facial edema)
- bronchial spasm.
- Musculoskeletal System Arthritis;
- arthralgia;
- myalgia.
- Nervous System Encephalitis;
- encephalopathy;
- measles inclusion body encephalitis (MIBE)
- subacute sclerosing panencephalitis (SSPE);
- Guillain-Barré Syndrome (GBS);
- acute disseminated encephalomyelitis (ADEM);
- transverse myelitis;
- febrile convulsions;
- afebrile convulsions or seizures;
- ataxia;
- polyneuritis;
- polyneuropathy;
- ocular palsies;
- paresthesia.
- Respiratory System Pneumonia;
- pneumonitis; sore throat;
- cough;

- rhinitis.
- Skin Stevens-Johnson syndrome;
- acute hemorrhagic edema of infancy;
- Henoch-Schönlein purpura;
- erythema multiforme;
- urticaria;
- rash;
- measles-like rash;
- pruritus;
- injection site reactions (pain, erythema, swelling and vesiculation).
- Ear Nerve deafness;
- otitis media.
- Eye Retinitis;
- optic neuritis;
- papillitis;
- conjunctivitis.
- Urogenital System Epididymitis;
- Orchitis

[A quick recap of side effects we saw earlier]

Two main things from this report about measles from Circleofmammas.com worth pointing out:

The range found among people groups, and how they differed compared to race and location, certainly aids in debunking the Germ Theory of disease. How can a "germ" differentiate between people groups, especially when they interact with each other? How can a "germ" care how much money a person makes, or how well off they are? All the statistics that have higher measles cases are related to a lack of cleanliness, means, crowded vs. uncrowded areas etc.

The other overwhelming factor was vaccination rates: with the vaccinated having much higher incidences.

**Two more stories:**

Toddler Dies 30 Hours After 3 Shots: MMR, Varicella and Hep A Vaccinations

February 20, 2024

*Shared from his mother, Gabriella.*

"Hi my name is Gabriella, the mother of Dino Angelo Santuccione, who lost his life at 1 years old due to vaccines.

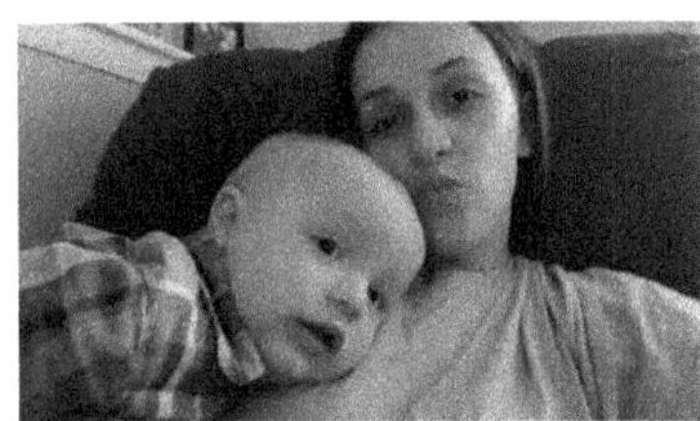

It was like any normal day I took him to his 1-year-old checkup appointment at Guilderland Pediatrician where my Son received 3 shots that day: MMR, VARICELLA, HEP A vaccines.

My baby boy did not show any signs concerning. He had a low-grade fever the night before his passing and his father administered Motrin and a hour later my baby boy went to bed, and did not wake up.

I lost my son 30 hours after he received his 1-year-old shots. My baby boy went into heart failure. When we found our son it was too late. And the police treated us like criminals and locked our house down for a few days, took our phones for 4 days, took my son's pillow he slept on, CPS investigated Nick and I and my 3 children and did not find anything suspicious!

We were plastered all over the news, Facebook, Newspaper, before they even investigated what happened to our baby boy.

My son was 32 pounds. Happy and healthy no issues, no abuse NO NOTHING! and CPS is blaming me because I did not go in and check on my baby boy in the middle of the night more!!!

We finally received news from a lawyer they want to take on our case because they have found something involving the vaccines that killed my son. My baby boy should still be here today and not forever be 1 years old because of these vaccines these doctors keep pushing on our baby's / children!

We have a voice, we should be able to stand up for our kids and what gets put into our babies' bodies'! I miss you so much Dino! It kills mommy, daddy and your sisters every day knowing you are not here with us anymore celebrating life. I miss your giggles and your huge warming smile, I miss your "WHATS THAT."

Sadly, the blaming and shaming of parents, to shift the spotlight from themselves, is an all-too-common occurrence in the medical profession where vaccines are concerned.

**"Measles Rash and 35-Minute Seizure 9 Days After Vaccines: Aiden's Story**

September 27, 2024

*Shared with permission from his mom:*

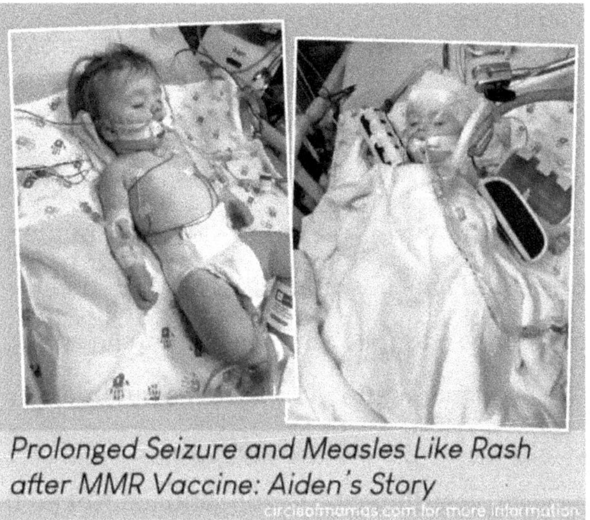


"This is my son Aiden after the MMR. He almost lost his life...never again.

Aiden received his MMR and 9 days later he broke out into a rash (measles) and the next day he randomly went unconscious on me in his high chair and a few minutes later started to have a seizure. His seizure lasted about 35 minutes until the hospital was finally able to stop it.

By the time the ambulance got him to the hospital his oxygen was at 9% as he was in hypoxia. I remember the doctor telling me that he isn't sure that my baby boy will make it but he is going to do everything he can to save him.  He was put on life support and when he was stable enough, he was transferred to a children's hospital.

The doctors eventually agreed this was a vaccine reaction. A day later he was able to come off of the ventilator by the grace of God!!! To go from almost losing his life to pulling through fully was a miracle.

I regret giving him any [vaccines] and will do whatever I can to spread awareness so other children and families do not have to go through what we have. Aiden did have another prolonged seizure and was hospitalized 2 months later.

We have, since, stopped vaccinating and he has been seizure free! He is on medication for seizures but hopefully can wean off of it soon and stay seizure free.

We are very, very lucky he is still with us. Not all families are.

He is 2 (almost 3) now. He had the MMR, Prevnar and Hepatitis. The reason we believe it was the MMR is because of all of his symptoms. He had the measles rash. They treated me well for the most part but after so many tests I believe they gave up and agreed it was a reaction to the vaccine."

Circle of Mammas goes on to state:

"I just want to express gratitude to Aiden's mom for sharing their story. Vaccines are such a contested topic, but people who experience vaccine reactions should not be mislabeled, mistreated, or denied their experience, just to maintain some illusion of safety. Let their voices be heard, and their stories be told.

We won't know exactly how rare or common vaccine reactions are because we stigmatize discussion and research into vaccine reactions. Several studies that investigated the health disparities of vaccinated and unvaccinated children concluded that unvaccinated children overall have fewer chronic conditions, such as neurodevelopment disorders and asthma.

Many studies that investigate the "safety of vaccination" fail to include a fully unvaccinated reference group or control, rendering their results useless, and non-applicable to the question: "Are vaccines associated with ____?" Only an "unexposed" comparator would be able to sufficiently answer that question.

In this case, Aiden developed a measles like rash after vaccination, and also a prolonged seizure–both validated and verified vaccine reactions according to the vaccine inserts. According to the MMR vaccine insert, which is a legal document where all possible side effects must be disclosed, around 6% or 9% of infants had different rashes, depending on injection route and concomitant administration, up to 42 days post-vaccination.

*"The nature of any rash was characterized by principal investigator either as measles-like, rubella-like, varicella-like or "other."*

These rashes are categorized as separate rashes, however in total, up to 9% of infants reported rashes. So, if the frequency is around 9% that is about 1 in 10 infants will develop some rash after the MMR vaccine.

| Solicited systemic reactions (Days 0 to 42) | | |
|---|---|---|
| Measles-like rash[§] | 2.9 | 2.7 |
| Rubella-like rash[§] | 2.7 | 2.7 |
| Varicella-like rash[§] | 0.5. | 3.2 |
| Mumps-like illness | 0 | 0.3 |
| Fever (temperature ≥38.0°C)[¶] [*] | 66.5 | 66.8 |
| 38.0-38.5°C | 20.4 | 22.2 |
| >38.5-39.0°C | 17.4 | 16.6 |
| >39.0-39.5°C | 14.2 | 13.4 |
| >39.5-40.0°C | 11.8 | 11.0 |
| >40.0°C | 2.7 | 3.7 |

Over 66% of the infants had a fever over ≥38.0°C which is (100.4°F).

I have a feeling there are far more of these reactions than is recognized. Some rashes are misdiagnosed (hand foot and mouth?), and some seizures are not witnessed, not recognized, not documented or not reported. Seizures, both febrile and afebrile, have a long history of being related to vaccination, including the MMR vaccines, as well as adjuvanted toxoid vaccines like DTP and DTaP.

**From the MMR vaccine insert:**

Nervous System

Encephalitis; encephalopathy; measles inclusion body encephalitis (MIBE) subacute sclerosing, panencephalitis (SSPE); Guillain-Barré Syndrome (GBS); acute disseminated encephalomyelitis (ADEM);

transverse myelitis; febrile convulsions; afebrile convulsions or seizures; ataxia; polyneuritis;

polyneuropathy; ocular palsies; paresthesia; syncope.

The frequency of seizures after MMR vaccine varies dependent on study design.

According to an unsourced sentence from the CDC:

*MMR vaccination has previously been associated with febrile seizures occurring 8-14 days after vaccination; among children aged <7 years, approximately* ***one additional febrile seizure occurs among every 3,000-4,000 children vaccinated with MMR vaccine,*** *compared with children not vaccinated during the preceding 30 days.*

A 2021 Geier and Geier longitudinal study reported: According to a 2014 population-based cohort study that looked at MMRV (rather than just MMR), the additional combination shot produced an additional seizure risk (in addition to the MMR+V):

*During the 7- to 10-day peak period, the risk of febrile seizures among children receiving their first dose of MMRV was double that for same-day administration of the separate vaccines. This translates to an additional 3.52 seizures per 10,000 doses administered, or 1 excess seizure for every 2841 doses administered.*

A 2019 paper looked at whether preterm and full-term infants have similar or different rates of seizure after MMR vaccine and MMRV vaccine. This is a VSD study, and they only looked at vaccinated infants.

*There were 532,375 children (45,343 preterm and 487,032 full-term) who received their first dose of measles-containing vaccine at age 12 through 23 months. The IRRs of febrile seizures*

*7 through 10 days compared with 15 through 42 days after receipt of measles-containing vaccine were 3.9 (95% CI: 2.5-6.0) in preterm children and 3.2 (2.7-3.7) in full-term children; the ratio of IRRs: was 1.2 (0.76-1.9), p = 0.41.*

If you read the full text, both the full term and premature infants had double the rate of seizure after MMRV than MMR. Without an unvaccinated comparator, we can't conclude much about MMR alone.

A 2021 Geier and Geier longitudinal study reported:

*The current study revealed that about 1 in 3,100 doses of MMR vaccine administered to children from 12 through 16 months of age are attributably associated with a seizure disorder diagnosis following an initial seizure episode with an onset of symptoms from 6 to 11 days post-MMR vaccination.*

*The daily incidence rate of an initial seizure episode diagnosed from 6 to 11 days post-MMR vaccination in comparison to 12 to17 months among unvaccinated persons was significantly increased (unadjusted HR = 5.73, p < 0.0001 and adjusted HR = 5.94, p < 0.0001) in HR models.*

*The observed rate of seizure disorder diagnosis post-MMR vaccination is estimated to be a > 80% reduction as compared to natural measles infection.*

In regard to the last sentence, it is based on a German paper written in 1925. Geier and Geier write:

*"By way of comparison, a previous study evaluated 5,940 cases of measles over a 25-year period for neurological*

*manifestations. A total of 11 children were diagnosed with seizure disorder (1 in 540 children). As a rough estimate, this means that the childhood MMR vaccination as compared to natural measles infection is associated with about a 6-fold reduction (>80% reduction) in the rate of seizure disorder diagnoses (MMR vaccine = 1 in 3,100 children vs natural measles infection = 1 in 540 children).*"

The Circle of Mammas website goes on to quote:

"Everyone born before 1963 had a natural measles infection. Did 1 in 540 of those generations have a seizure disorder? We would need more research, including capturing subclinical measles infections, to gauge what the actual neurological risks to natural measles infection are, *in a society that isn't confounded with other toxins that can cause neurological issues*, IE. other vaccines, pesticides, poisons, etc. The paper is in German and looked at children born prior to 1925. Children in the first decades of the 1900s were routinely given poisons as "medicinal" nostrums, cordials, elixirs and powders, simply because we didn't know better. Chloroform was used to stop convulsions.

In 1911, the treatment for measles as recommended here was carbolic oil (phenol), which is a coal derivative, highly poisonous, and causes convulsions and death. It was advised to rub it on a child's tonsils and throat. So no. I cannot entertain such insanity when I know that the Victorian era and the Edwardian era was marked by patent medicines made using dangerous elemental concoctions such as mercury, lead and arsenic that poisoned and killed. The conclusions from a 1925 paper would be confounded by all the medications used routinely in that era and there is no way we can prove which caused what, and whether measles was responsible for the sequelae, or the contemporaneous medical interventions used to "treat" measles. I'm not even mentioning the measles immune globulin that was administered with a reused, unsterilized syringe and needle. How did that section of the paper pass peer review?

The only part of that paper I am privy to:

*"Some remarkable cases of nervous side effects and sequelae in acute infectious diseases of childhood stimulated the attempt to give an overview of what has been observed so far in this area. For this purpose, in addition to a compilation of the relevant literature, I have subjected the rich medical history material of our institution, the Kaiser and Kaiser in Friedrich Children's Hospital in Berlin, to a more detailed review. 5,940 cases of measles (born 1905-1925), 2,690 cases of whooping cough (1911-1925) and 2,440 cases of scarlet fever (1915-1925) were examined to determine the extent to which complications from the nervous system could be identified during the course of or following the diseases mentioned."*

Sorry, but I am shocked these authors think this study can relate to today's children experiencing a natural measles infection. There is literally a paper from 1895 titled "*Measles and Phenacetin: Which Killed the Patient-The Disease or the*

*Treatment*" because there was an inkling even back then that medications can be a toxic response to a mostly benign infection in a well-nourished person.

But I do have a question, since that German paper looked for nervous system manifestations post viral infection in children and followed them for many years: *How many of the children developed autism?*

Which would have been impossible to miss, am I right?

Today, 1 in 36 children are on the Autism spectrum, and in California it's 1 in 22. Many of these children are non-verbal, hand flapping, head banging, fitting and tantruming. Some are still in diapers. And yes, children with autism have a higher risk of a seizure disorder. So again, my question, how many of the children with nervous system disorders in Germany in the early 1900s who experienced a measles or scarlet fever infection and were monitored for years went on to develop autism, a good 20 years before Leo Kanner would even be the first to describe the condition?

The true toll of vaccines like the MMR vaccine is unknown because <u>no one</u> is doing robust, complete, bias-free surveillance and few parents are aware of the Vaccine Adverse Event Reporting System (VAERS)–however, there is *no deadline* to report." (see link to full article in the Appendix sect.)

The majority of this particular report was to prove that the "so-called studies" that medical journals and physicians and those trying to advocate for vaccines, reference, in an attempt to declare the "proof" that vaccines are less dangerous than disease, are too old and during a time period when other treatments being widely used to treat such cases were heavily toxic and not being accounted for, as well as the fact that the data sighted was all about proving MMR was less violent in creating seizures and other adverse reactions than a cocktail that contained one extra vaccine. Glancing at the report on NIH, I'm surprised that no one is mentioning the fact that only the 6-11th days post MMR initial dose was monitored or recorded vs. birth through 16 mo. for unvaccinated with no regard for any other possible contaminants, (including DPT or other vaccines?) This most certainly is NOT a reliable study to prove any safety or efficacy of the MMR or other vaccine. This is the largest problem, though with all the "safety studies" that have been done: none of them are actually scientifically sound or unbiased comparisons of vaccinated to unvaccinated. For the same reasons that vaccines must be categorized as "unavoidably unsafe" no authentic or comprehensive analysis can be done or it would prove the inefficacy and danger of vaccines.

## Conclusions of the MMR Vaccine:

It would be a vast understatement to say that the measles vaccine has been shown to cause substantially more damage than any natural case of measles ever reported, honestly. An outbreak of measles (keep in mind it is a detox reaction), for typical ("natural") reasons, only ever caused death in places where living conditions were fatal or other issues were present. The adjuvants alone in the MMR vaccine, pose a far more serious threat than any natural infection. It is a fact, that the amount of vaccine damage recognized by the medical field is such a small percentage of actual cases. This is a reason I include the stories as they are the only definitive and observable record of real damage.

Any "protection" a vaccine could possibly offer does not last (this is stated even by those who advocate for vaccines) and could be a cause of getting the disease when otherwise there would have been no exposure.

Truly, the fate of your child as well as the future of your family and those of future generations would be better served by going to "measles outbreak parties" then by allowing your child to be injected with these known toxins. I don't believe any of that is necessary (and will talk more about why later) but **anything** you can do to strengthen the body's immune system or increase nutrition or cleanliness would impact your child's health (for good) a hundredfold more than any vaccine ever could.

This is not the only section we talk about the MMR vaccine, specifically, and at the time of writing of this book, the MMR has seen a resurgence of attention. Voices like those of Dell Bigtree, RFK, and multitudes in the mainstream medical circles are discussing a renewed push for getting people to take this vaccine. Much that we discuss in several of the stories, the chapters on *The Science* and *What is a Virus* and more in the Appendix contain vital information for understanding why this vaccine (along with the others) is one of the worst things you could push in attempts to irradicate the disease.

## VIT. K

The vitamin K shot is one of the earliest pushed injections for newborns and may seem like one of the few necessary ones. At least that is how I viewed it for many years. Yet, it is not as necessary or safe as they try to make it sound. For the last baby I had (which is only 6 months ago at the time of my writing this), I actually never realized that the Vit.K shot they recommend (even for preemies) contains Aluminum. Though they tell you it's such a teeny, tiny amount, and the syringe is one of the smallest administered, how is any aluminum a good idea or safe for babies? I asked about the oral option, but apparently, it is not one they keep on hand as they do the injection.

The first bit of information I want to share on here, came from a variety of sources: a post from Innate Doula Services, Merck & Co's own data, packaging inserts, etc.

"It is a well-known fact that newborns are born with low Vitamin K. As in every instance, God has a reason for this. One reason that has been discovered is that a baby's cord blood is full of stem cells that can be utilized for quick healing to areas that may experience trauma, even during the labor and delivery process. As the cord is still full of these precious cells at birth, it is a reason for delaying cord clamping immediately after birth (especially while the cord is still pulsating). If Vitamin K levels were higher, it would slow the process of these vital cells arriving speedily where most needed." It is also worth noting that the grave concern of brain hemorrhage has only occurred in less than 2% of babies. It is impossible to know whether these were even directly related to low Vit.K levels or another complication.

What one must truly wonder is why the Vit.K shot is so highly recommended when it contains known toxins to humans and an oral vitamin K would be more effective, without any of the toxins contained in the shot.

Just take a look at the warning on the label:

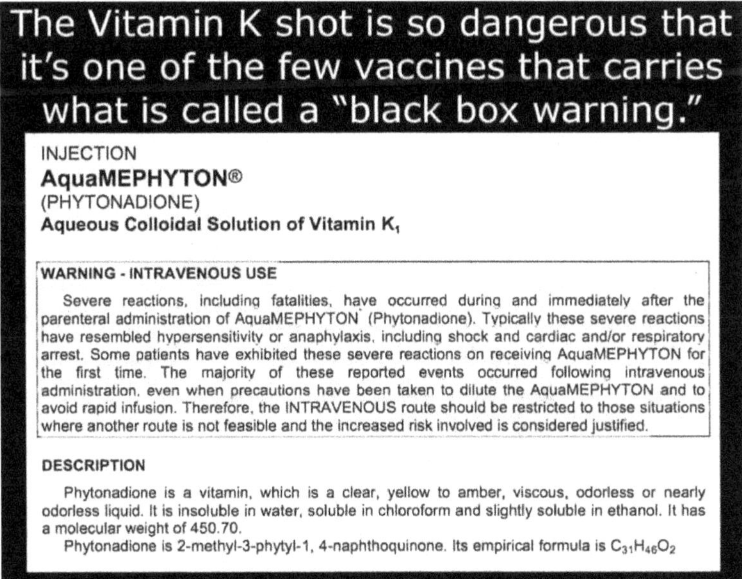

The Vitamin K shot is so dangerous that it's one of the few vaccines that carries what is called a "black box warning."

INJECTION

**AquaMEPHYTON®**

(PHYTONADIONE)

**Aqueous Colloidal Solution of Vitamin $K_1$**

**WARNING - INTRAVENOUS USE**

Severe reactions, including fatalities, have occurred during and immediately after the parenteral administration of AquaMEPHYTON (Phytonadione). Typically these severe reactions have resembled hypersensitivity or anaphylaxis, including shock and cardiac and/or respiratory arrest. Some patients have exhibited these severe reactions on receiving AquaMEPHYTON for the first time. The majority of these reported events occurred following intravenous administration, even when precautions have been taken to dilute the AquaMEPHYTON and to avoid rapid infusion. Therefore, the INTRAVENOUS route should be restricted to those situations where another route is not feasible and the increased risk involved is considered justified.

**DESCRIPTION**

Phytonadione is a vitamin, which is a clear, yellow to amber, viscous, odorless or nearly odorless liquid. It is insoluble in water, soluble in chloroform and slightly soluble in ethanol. It has a molecular weight of 450.70.

Phytonadione is 2-methyl-3-phytyl-1, 4-naphthoquinone. Its empirical formula is $C_{31}H_{46}O_2$

The following is copied from the actual insert of the Vit. K intramuscular injection, look at the warnings and contraindications:

**VITAMIN K INJECTION**
**Phytonadione**
**Injectable Emulsion, USP**
®N+
**Aqueous Dispersion of Vitamin K**
**Ampul**
**Rx only**
**Protect from light. Keep ampuls in tray until time of use.**
**WARNING – INTRAVENOUS AND INTRAMUSCULAR USE**

Severe reactions, including fatalities, have occurred during and immediately after INTRAVENOUS injection of phytonadione, even when precautions have been taken to dilute the phytonadione and to avoid rapid infusion. Severe reactions, including fatalities, have also been reported following INTRAMUSCULAR administration. Typically these severe reactions have resembled hypersensitivity or anaphylaxis, including shock and cardiac and/or respiratory arrest. Some patients have exhibited these severe reactions on receiving phytonadione for the first time. Therefore the INTRAVENOUS and INTRAMUSCULAR routes should be restricted to those situations where the subcutaneous route is not feasible and the serious risk involved is considered justified.

**DESCRIPTION**

Phytonadione is a vitamin, which is a clear, yellow to amber, viscous, odorless or nearly odorless liquid. It is insoluble in water, soluble in chloroform and slightly soluble in ethanol. It has a molecular weight of 450.70.

Phytonadione is 2methyl3phytyl1, 4naphthoquinone.

Its empirical formula is C H O and its structural formula is:

Vitamin K Injection (Phytonadione Injectable Emulsion, USP) is a yellow, sterile, nonpyrogenic aqueous dispersion available for

injection by the intravenous, intramuscular and subcutaneous routes. Each milliliter contains phytonadione 2 or 10 mg,

polyoxyethylated fatty acid derivative 70 mg, dextrose, hydrous 37.5 mg in water for injection; benzyl alcohol 9 mg added as

preservative. May contain hydrochloric acid for pH adjustment. pH is 6.3 (5.0 to 7.0). Phytonadione is oxygen sensitive.

**CONTRAINDICATION**

Hypersensitivity to any component of this medication.

**WARNINGS**

Benzyl alcohol as a preservative in Bacteriostatic Sodium Chloride Injection has been associated with toxicity in newborns. Data is unavailable on the toxicity of other preservatives in this age group. There is no evidence to suggest that the small amount of benzyl alcohol contained in Vitamin K Injection (Phytonadione Injectable Emulsion, USP), when used as recommended, is associated with toxicity.

An immediate coagulant effect should not be expected after administration of phytonadione. It takes a minimum of 1 to 2 hours for measurable improvement in the prothrombin time. Whole blood or component therapy may also be necessary if bleeding is severe.

Phytonadione will not counteract the anticoagulant action of heparin.

When vitamin K is used to correct excessive anticoagulant induced hypoprothrombinemia, anticoagulant therapy still being indicated, the patient is again faced with the clotting hazards existing prior to starting the anticoagulant therapy. Phytonadione is not a clotting agent, but overzealous therapy with vitamin K may restore conditions which originally permitted thromboembolic phenomena. Dosage should be kept as low as possible, and prothrombin time should be checked regularly as clinical conditions indicate.

Repeated large doses of vitamin K are not warranted in liver disease if the response to initial use of the vitamin is unsatisfactory. Failure to respond to vitamin K may indicate that the condition being treated is inherently unresponsive to vitamin K.

Benzyl alcohol has been reported to be associated with a fatal "Gasping Syndrome" in premature infants.

WARNING: This product contains aluminum that may be toxic. Aluminum may reach toxic levels with prolonged parenteral administration if kidney function is impaired. Premature neonates are particularly at risk because their kidneys are immature, and they require large amounts of calcium and phosphate solutions, which contain aluminum.

Research indicates that patients with impaired kidney function, including premature neonates, who receive parenteral levels of aluminum at greater than 4 to 5 mcg/kg/day accumulate aluminum at levels associated with central nervous system and bone toxicity.

Tissue loading may occur at even lower rates of administration.

**PRECAUTIONS**

**Drug Interactions**

Temporary resistance to prothrombin depressing anticoagulants may result, especially when larger doses of phytonadione are used. If relatively large doses have been employed, it may be necessary when reinstituting anticoagulant therapy to use somewhat larger doses of the prothrombin depressing anticoagulant, or to use one which acts on a different principle, such as heparin sodium.

**Laboratory Tests**

Prothrombin time should be checked regularly as clinical conditions indicate.

**Carcinogenesis, Mutagenesis, Impairment of Fertility**

Studies of carcinogenicity, mutagenesis or impairment of fertility have not been conducted with Vitamin K Injection (Phytonadione Injectable Emulsion, USP).

**Pregnancy**

Pregnancy Category C

Animal reproduction studies have not been conducted with Vitamin K Injection. It is also not known whether Vitamin K Injection can cause fetal harm when administered to a pregnant woman or can affect reproduction capacity. Vitamin K Injection should be given to a pregnant woman only if clearly needed.

**Nursing Mothers**

It is not known whether this drug is excreted in human milk. Because many drugs are excreted in human milk, caution should be exercised when Vitamin K Injection is administered to a nursing woman.

**Pediatric Use**

Hemolysis, jaundice, and hyperbilirubinemia in neonates, particularly those that are premature, may be related to the dose of Vitamin K Injection. Therefore, the recommended dose should not be exceeded (see ADVERSE REACTIONS and DOSAGE AND ADMINISTRATION).

**ADVERSE REACTIONS**

Deaths have occurred after intravenous and intramuscular administration. (See Box Warning.)

Transient "flushing sensations" and "peculiar" sensations of taste have been observed, as well as rare instances of dizziness, rapid and weak pulse, profuse sweating, brief hypotension, dyspnea, and cyanosis.

Pain, swelling, and tenderness at the injection site may occur.

The possibility of allergic sensitivity including an anaphylactoid reaction, should be kept in mind.

Infrequently, usually after repeated injection, erythematous, indurated, pruritic plaques have occurred; rarely, these have progressed to scleroderma like lesions that have persisted for long periods. In other cases, these lesions have resembled erythema perstans.

Hyperbilirubinemia has been observed in the newborn following administration of phytonadione. This has occurred rarely and primarily with doses above those recommended. (See PRECAUTIONS, Pediatric Use.)

I find it rather astounding that Hemolysis (which is destruction of red blood cells) and Hyperbilirubinemia (which would naturally follow) are possible reactions of the Vit. K shot, which is recommended to prevent possible bleeding and hemorrhaging. Particularly, in my baby's case, since excessive bilirubin is what my baby was being hospitalized for, yet they were pushing for the vit. K injection, despite all the possible contraindications, for a possible brain bleed issue that occurs in less than 2% of newborns.

Traditionally, Israelis circumcise their children on the 8th day after birth, which, consequently, is when Vit. K is naturally at its peak. If you want to have this procedure done in the hospital, or later, the safest option for your baby, would simply be to wait until the baby is ready.

There are multiple ways to raise Vit. K levels naturally if that is a concern. A mom eating foods high in Vit.K (such as green, leafy vegetables) before giving birth would increase baby's levels. So would after birth if mom is nursing. Colostrum, itself, is naturally high in Vit. K. If there is a further need or recommendation, taking an oral dose should not be a problem for your doctor to consider.

If more parents were informed and spoke out on this issue, hospitals and doctors would be forced to change their policies and recommendations.

# HEP. B

I am sorry to say, I have had this injection myself, since it was required before I was allowed to do clinicals at the hospital where I was studying nursing at the time. As those who have had it know, it is scheduled in 3 doses.

The greatest danger of this vaccine is harm to infants, especially since it is one of the first recommended for them. There is now information, including history of the disease, to show that the profound damage and symptoms associated with "viral hepatitis" (which is really inflammation of the liver, attributed to said virus) was always due to medications and drugs, extremely poor diet, certain life-style choices, as well as a number of other possible things that damage the liver or cause inflammation. Most often, medications and drugs. I will talk more about this in the section on VIRUSES.

## Adverse Reactions:

This is taken from the insert of a HB vaccine. Keep in mind, this is only a small fraction of damage occurring from vaccine administration.

"In a group of studies, 3258 doses of RECOMBIVAX HB, 10 mcg, were administered to 1252 healthy adults who were monitored for 5 days after each dose. Injection site reactions and systemic adverse reactions were reported following 17% and

15% of the injections, respectively. The following adverse reactions were reported: Incidence Equal To or Greater Than 1% of Injections

GENERAL DISORDERS AND ADMINISTRATION SITE CONDITIONS

Injection site reactions consisting principally of soreness, and including pain, tenderness, pruritus, erythema, ecchymosis, swelling, warmth, nodule formation. The most frequent systemic complaints include fatigue/weakness; headache; fever (≥100°F); malaise.

GASTROINTESTINAL DISORDERS Nausea; diarrhea

RESPIRATORY, THORACIC AND MEDIASTINAL DISORDERS Pharyngitis; upper respiratory infection Incidence Less Than 1% of Injections

GENERAL DISORDERS AND ADMINISTRATION SITE CONDITIONS Sweating; achiness; sensation of warmth; lightheadedness; chills; flushing

GASTROINTESTINAL DISORDERS Vomiting; abdominal pains/cramps; dyspepsia; diminished appetite RESPIRATORY, THORACIC AND MEDIASTINAL DISORDERS Rhinitis; influenza; cough

NERVOUS SYSTEM DISORDERS Vertigo/dizziness; paresthesia

SKIN AND SUBCUTANEOUS TISSUE DISORDERS Pruritus; rash (non-specified); angioedema; urticaria MUSCULOSKELETAL AND CONNECTIVE TISSUE DISORDERS Arthralgia including monoarticular; myalgia; back pain; neck pain; shoulder pain; neck stiffness

BLOOD AND LYMPHATIC DISORDERS Lymphadenopathy

PSYCHIATRIC DISORDERS Insomnia/disturbed sleep

EAR AND LABYRINTH DISORDERS Earache

RENAL AND URINARY DISORDERS Dysuria

CARDIAC DISORDERS Hypotension

## Post-Marketing Experience

The following additional adverse reactions have been reported with use of the marketed vaccine. Because these reactions are reported voluntarily from a population of uncertain size, it is not possible to reliably estimate their frequency or establish a causal relationship to a vaccine exposure.

Immune System Disorders Hypersensitivity reactions including anaphylactic/anaphylactoid reactions, bronchospasm, and urticaria have been reported within the first few hours after vaccination. An apparent hypersensitivity syndrome (serum-sickness-like) of delayed onset has been reported days to weeks after vaccination, including: arthralgia/arthritis (usually transient), fever, and dermatologic reactions such as urticaria, erythema multiforme, ecchymoses and erythema nodosum [see Warnings and Precautions (5.1)].

Autoimmune diseases including systemic lupus erythematosus (SLE), lupus-like syndrome, vasculitis, and polyarteritis nodosa have also been reported.

Gastrointestinal Disorders Elevation of liver enzymes; constipation

Nervous System Disorders Guillain-Barré syndrome; multiple sclerosis; exacerbation of multiple sclerosis; myelitis including transverse myelitis; seizure; febrile seizure; peripheral neuropathy including Bell's Palsy; radiculopathy; herpes zoster; migraine; muscle weakness; hypesthesia; encephalitis

Skin and Subcutaneous Disorders Stevens-Johnson syndrome; alopecia; petechiae; eczema Musculoskeletal and Connective Tissue Disorders Arthritis Pain in extremity

Blood and Lymphatic System Disorders Increased erythrocyte sedimentation rate; thrombocytopenia Psychiatric Disorders Irritability; agitation; somnolence

Eye Disorders Optic neuritis; tinnitus; conjunctivitis; visual disturbances; uveitis

Cardiac Disorders Syncope; tachycardia"

Oh yes, and we need to add, DEATH to that list.

## Another Story from Circle of Mammas

February 17, 2025

"My letter to Nicole Shanahan:

Hi Nicole,

I felt compelled to reach out to you as a fellow vaccine injury mom. I want to share the story of our daughter, Caroline "Charlee" Baker.

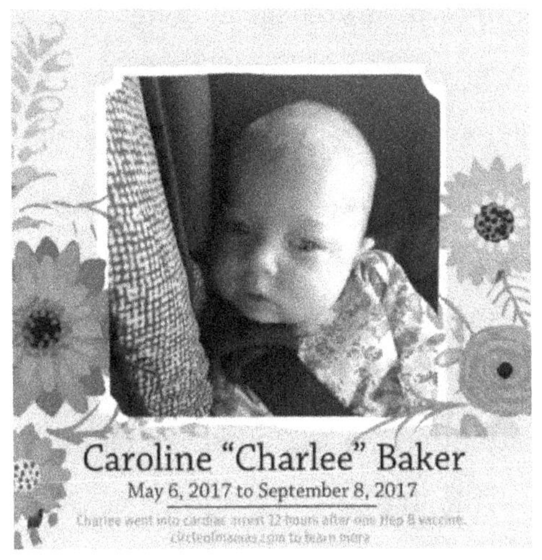


Charlee was born on May 6, 2017, after an unremarkable pregnancy. She was delivered via C-section, weighing 6 lbs 8 oz. We declined the Hep B vaccine at the hospital, preferring to have our own pediatrician administer it.

At 18 days old, she received the **Recombivax Hep B vaccine**. She had been thriving—nursing well, gaining weight, and was such a content little girl.

But 22 hours later, everything changed.

Charlee suffered a sudden cardiac arrest while nursing—she just stopped. I was at Panera with a colleague, both of us Certified Registered Nurse Anesthesiologists with neonatal and pediatric experience. By some miracle, we were able to resuscitate her, but she suffered a severe anoxic brain injury, leading to a two-month stay at Children's Hospital of Detroit—where I was employed as a staff nurse anesthesiologist at the time.

She had a million-dollar workup, but not one doctor would acknowledge that the vaccine could have caused her cardiac arrest. Genetic testing for her, my husband, and me all came back negative.

At two months old, as she was preparing to be discharged, doctors wanted to give her more vaccines. I didn't know what I know now, but I knew enough to insist that she be on a cardiac monitor during them. She received Hib and Prevnar, and immediately after, she went into bradycardia and apnea.

At that moment, my husband and I knew—the vaccines had caused this.

A neonatologist even admitted the "quiet part out loud," saying she routinely tells residents to put the crash cart next to NICU isolates when babies receive vaccines.

Charlee died suddenly at 4 months and 2 days old, in the middle of the night.

We have a case in the Vaccine Injury Compensation Program (VICP), but Special Master Nora Beth Dorsey *has already indicated she will rule against us*. She, like so many others, is captured by the pharmaceutical industry.

Since losing Charlee, we have been blessed with two boys—her little brothers—both completely unvaccinated and 100% healthy. While their friends and classmates struggle with asthma, food allergies, autism, chronic ear infections, and other now common childhood "illnesses," my boys have had none of these issues. They are thriving, strong, and healthy in a way that is impossible to ignore.

Our case: 1:19-vv-01327 – BAKER et al v. SECRETARY OF HEALTH AND HUMAN SERVICES

https://www.govinfo.gov/.../USCOURTS-cofc-1_19-vv.../summary

Special Master Nora Beth Dorsey:
https://www.uscfc.uscourts.gov/nora-beth-dorsey

When we file VICP cases, we are actually suing the Secretary of HHS, and now, that position belongs to your former running mate, RFK Jr. This is our hail Mary. We want some form of justice for our little girl.

As a mother, I know you understand the deep suffering of losing a child to a corrupt system. Thank you for taking the time to read this and thank you for all you are doing for our children and our country.

With gratitude,

Sarah Baker, MS, CRNA"

Many parents' pleas for justice can take years without seeing any resolution. The frustration they experience with government stipulations and hospital denial while grieving the loss of their child is beyond heart-wrenching.

Please believe me when I say that the stories about these vaccine damaged kids and the devastation of their families are a small percentage of the reality. Any adverse reactions you can find on the internet represents a small portion of the reality.

Another Story:

Preemie Dies Two Weeks After Delayed 'Well Baby' Visit

January 31, 2025

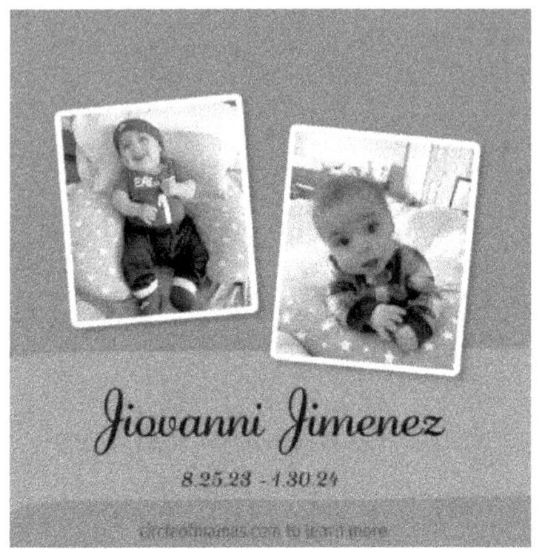


Jiovanni Jimenez was born at 35 weeks on August 25, 2023, weighing just 5 pounds 2 ounces. Despite the fact he was born premature, little Jiovanni was so healthy he overcame the NICU in just three days, according to his mom, Heather Biesel. By the time Jiovanni reached two months old, he was already in the 70% percentile for weight and growth.

Due to scheduling conflicts, Jiovanni's four-month shots were delayed closer to five months.

*"He did not like to take the [oral vaccine] well when they inserted he spit it up and they wanted to give more and I said 'No.' Thirteen days later my son passed."*

*"They linked it to SIDS, but I will never not believe it was vaccine related. I watched him drool and get fussier more and at the time I linked it to teething. I will regret it every day."*

According to Heather, the medical examiner did the bare minimum due to work load.

*"I fought for them to even complete their job and move him to the funeral home. They left it 'Undetermined.' I then called multiple times for them to give me reasoning."*

*"And they said no reason could put weight over another, which was insane to me. But they told me they needed to examine*

*every organ from heart to brain which affected his body and me preparing him for his funeral. No organ showed signs of illness or heaviness."*

Perfectly healthy before getting the vaccines, and growing beautifully, Jiovanni passed away suddenly on January 30, 2024, just 13 days after getting the CDC recommended vaccines.

Now, Jiovanni's mom is a warrior, bravely telling her son's story and blowing the whistle on Sudden Infant Death Syndrome. She won't be following the rules anymore, she said.

*"I know what I know and will fight for other moms as well."*

Obviously, this baby received more than the Hep. B vaccine, but that is most often the case.

What exactly does the CDC recommend?

Note: All these can be found on the CDCs website.

For 2023

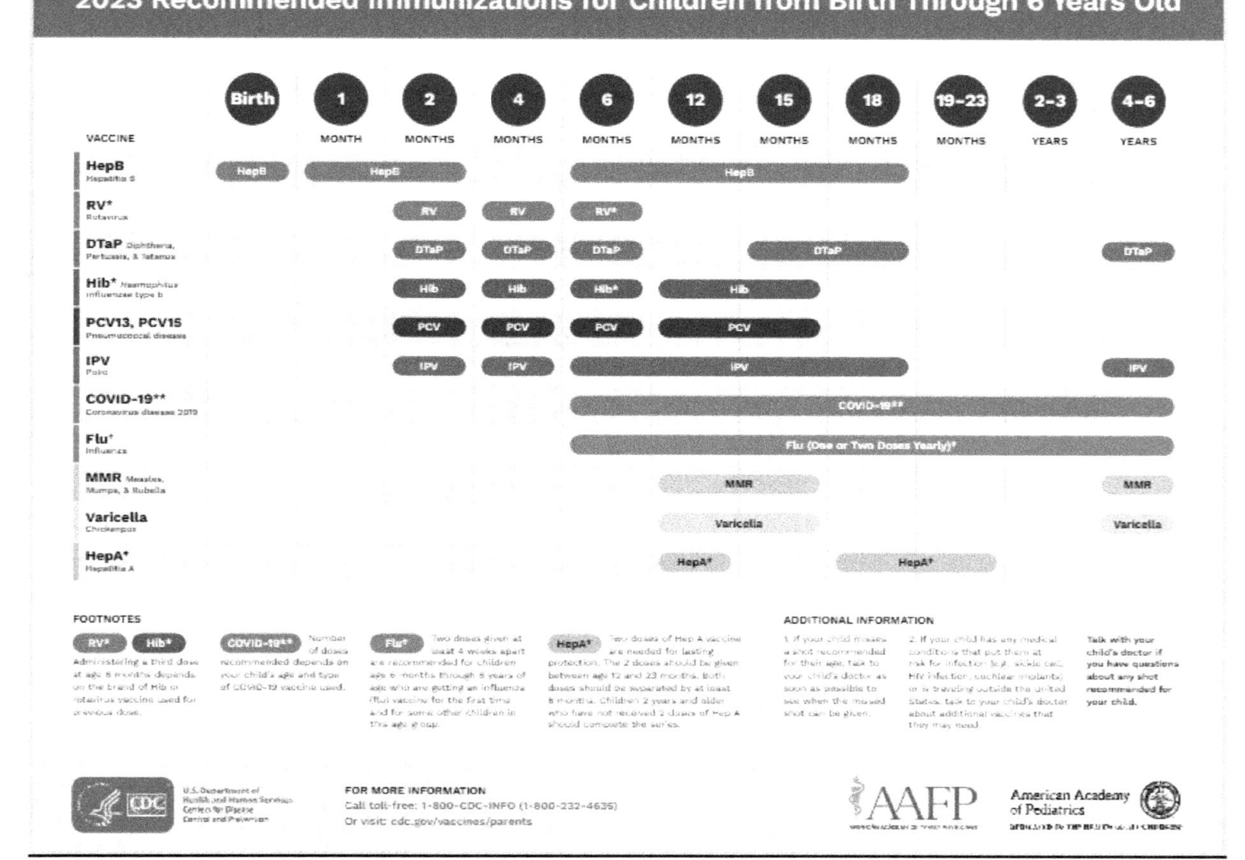
2023 Recommended Immunizations for Children from Birth Through 6 Years Old
VACCINE
Birth
1 MONTH
2 MONTHS
4 MONTHS
6 MONTHS
12 MONTHS
15 MONTHS
18 MONTHS
19–23 MONTHS
2–3 YEARS
4–6 YEARS
HepB Hepatitis B
HepB
HepB
HepB
RV* Rotavirus
RV
RV
RV*
DTaP Diphtheria, Pertussis, & Tetanus
DTaP
DTaP
DTaP
DTaP
DTaP
Hib* Haemophilus influenzae type b
Hib
Hib
Hib*
Hib
PCV13, PCV15 Pneumococcal disease
PCV
PCV
PCV
PCV
IPV Polio
IPV
IPV
IPV
IPV
COVID-19** Coronavirus disease 2019
COVID-19**
Flu* Influenza
Flu (One or Two Doses Yearly)*
MMR Measles, Mumps, & Rubella
MMR
MMR
Varicella Chickenpox
Varicella
Varicella
HepA* Hepatitis A
HepA*
HepA*
FOOTNOTES
RV* Hib* Administering a third dose at age 6 months depends on the brand of Hib or rotavirus vaccine used for previous dose.
COVID-19** Number of doses recommended depends on your child's age and type of COVID-19 vaccine used.
Flu* Two doses given at least 4 weeks apart are recommended for children age 6 months through 8 years of age who are getting an influenza (flu) vaccine for the first time and for some other children in this age group.
HepA* Two doses of Hep A vaccine are needed for lasting protection. The 2 doses should be given between age 12 and 23 months. Both doses should be separated by at least 6 months. Children 2 years and older who have not received 2 doses of Hep A should complete the series.
ADDITIONAL INFORMATION
1. If your child misses a shot recommended for their age, talk to your child's doctor as soon as possible to see when the missed shot can be given.
2. If your child has any medical conditions that put them at risk for infection (e.g., sickle cell, HIV infection, cochlear implants) or is traveling outside the United States, talk to your child's doctor about additional vaccines that they may need.
Talk with your child's doctor if you have questions about any shot recommended for your child.
U.S. Department of Health and Human Services
Centers for Disease Control and Prevention
FOR MORE INFORMATION
Call toll-free: 1-800-CDC-INFO (1-800-232-4636)
Or visit: cdc.gov/vaccines/parents
AAFP
American Academy of Pediatrics

For 2025

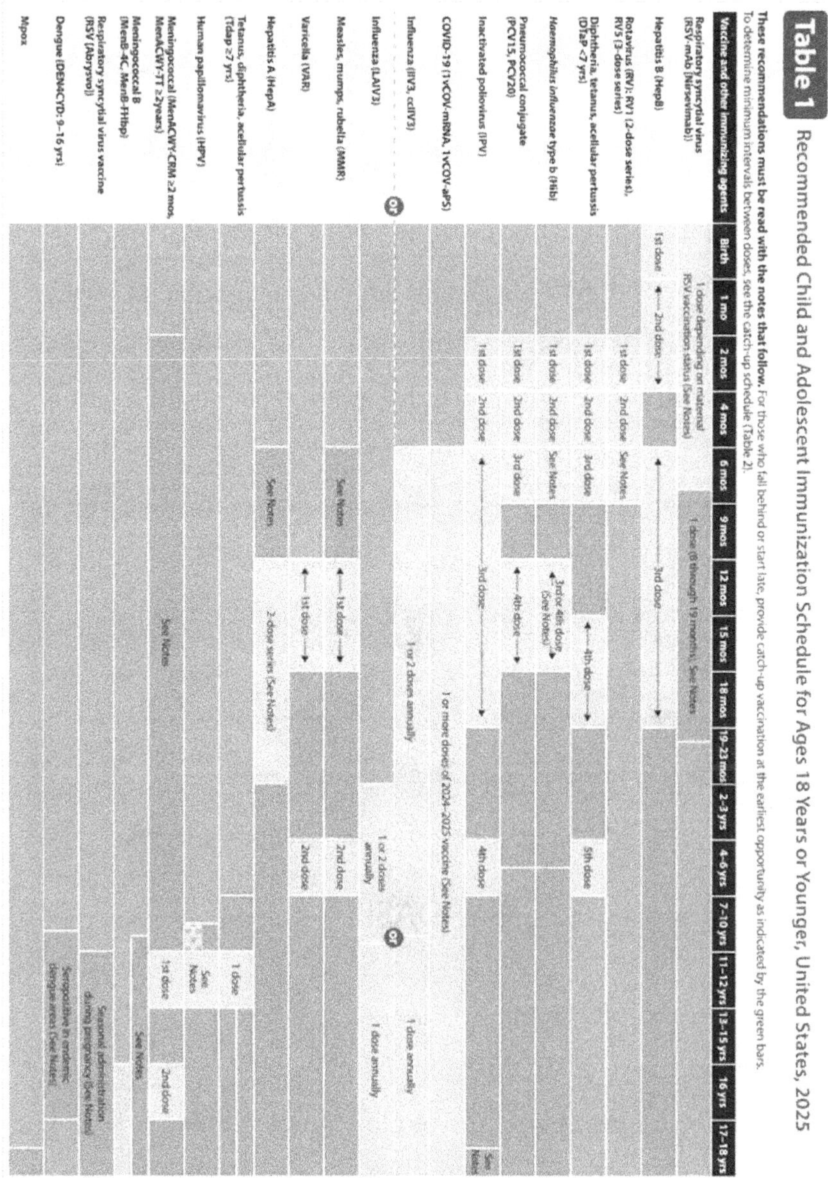

**Table 1** Recommended Child and Adolescent Immunization Schedule for Ages 18 Years or Younger, United States, 2025

**These recommendations must be read with the notes that follow.** For those who fall behind or start late, provide catch-up vaccination at the earliest opportunity as indicated by the green bars. To determine minimum intervals between doses, see the catch-up schedule (Table 2).

| Vaccine and other immunizing agents | Birth | 1 mo | 2 mos | 4 mos | 6 mos | 9 mos | 12 mos | 15 mos | 18 mos | 19–23 mos | 2–3 yrs | 4–6 yrs | 7–10 yrs | 11–12 yrs | 13–15 yrs | 16 yrs | 17–18 yrs |
|---|---|---|---|---|---|---|---|---|---|---|---|---|---|---|---|---|---|
| Respiratory syncytial virus (RSV-mAb [Nirsevimab]) | 1 dose depending on maternal RSV vaccination status (See Notes) | | | | | 1 dose (8 through 19 months), See Notes | | | | | | | | | | | |
| Hepatitis B (HepB) | 1st dose | ← 2nd dose → | | | ← 3rd dose → | | | | | | | | | | | | |
| Rotavirus (RV): RV1 (2-dose series), RV5 (3-dose series) | | | 1st dose | 2nd dose | See Notes | | | | | | | | | | | | |
| Diphtheria, tetanus, acellular pertussis (DTaP <7 yrs) | | | 1st dose | 2nd dose | 3rd dose | | | ← 4th dose → | | | | 5th dose | | | | | |
| *Haemophilus influenzae* type b (Hib) | | | 1st dose | 2nd dose | See Notes | | ← 3rd or 4th dose (See Notes) → | | | | | | | | | | |
| Pneumococcal conjugate (PCV15, PCV20) | | | 1st dose | 2nd dose | 3rd dose | | ← 4th dose → | | | | | | | | | | |
| Inactivated poliovirus (IPV) | | | 1st dose | 2nd dose | ← 3rd dose → | | | | | | | 4th dose | | | | | See Notes |
| COVID-19 (1vCOV-mRNA, 1vCOV-aPS) | | | | | 1 or more doses of 2024–2025 vaccine (See Notes) | | | | | | | | | | | | |
| Influenza (IIV3, ccIIV3) | | | | | 1 or 2 doses annually | | | | | | | | | | 1 dose annually | | |
| or | | | | | | | | | | | | | or | | | | |
| Influenza (LAIV3) | | | | | | | | | | | | 1 or 2 doses annually | | | 1 dose annually | | |
| Measles, mumps, rubella (MMR) | | | | | See Notes | | ← 1st dose → | | | | | 2nd dose | | | | | |
| Varicella (VAR) | | | | | | | ← 1st dose → | | | | | 2nd dose | | | | | |
| Hepatitis A (HepA) | | | | | See Notes | | 2-dose series (See Notes) | | | | | | | | | | |
| Tetanus, diphtheria, acellular pertussis (Tdap ≥7 yrs) | | | | | | | | | | | | | | 1 dose | | | |
| Human papillomavirus (HPV) | | | | | | | | | | | | | | See Notes | | | |
| Meningococcal (MenACWY-CRM ≥2 mos, MenACWY-TT ≥2years) | | | See Notes | | | | | | | | | | | 1st dose | | 2nd dose | |
| Meningococcal B (MenB-4C, MenB-FHbp) | | | | | | | | | | | | | | | | See Notes | |
| Respiratory syncytial virus vaccine (RSV [Abrysvo]) | | | | | | | | | | | | | | | | Seasonal administration during pregnancy (See Notes) | |
| Dengue (DEN4CYD: 9–16 yrs) | | | | | | | | | | | | | | | Seropositive in endemic dengue areas (See Notes) | | |
| Mpox | | | | | | | | | | | | | | | | | |

It is rather apparent that they are not planning on reducing the recommended number of vaccines. Hep B is one of the few vaccines recommended from birth and beyond. Since

Hepatitis B is an infection that has been known to be found in adults and passed on through intercourse and contaminated needles, one might wonder why infect, or bother preventing, if that were possible, in a newborn infant? The reasoning is that an infected mother could somehow pass it on to her child (I do not believe that is how liver disease can be acquired). The argument is wrapped around their claim that vaccination is responsible for keeping the Hep. B virus and others at bay.

It's Not. They rightfully point out that Hepatitis B is only problematic in countries with severe environmental and other conditions that contribute to the liver disease associated with the Hep. B virus. They wrongly credit vaccines for influencing (in any positive way) this reality. (but we will talk about this more in the THEORY section)

I'm not going to attempt to cover every recommended vaccine in depth, but we will talk about one more.

## GARDASIL

From a fellow Mom:

"If you have a daughter approaching the age of 12-14, she will soon be adamantly encouraged, by the attending nurse at her school, and by your very own family doctor, when you are out of the office, to receive the Gardasil HPV (human papillomavirus) vaccine, behind your back.

(I told Serahn to call me from school and run out of the gates so I could pick her up. No way that we were allowing this into her).

Inexplicably, this dangerous vaccine contains L-histidine, an essential amino acid, which plays a vital role in pregnancy; the synthetic form of which can also pass through the placental wall to the fetus. This could be the direct cause to the spontaneous miscarriage and birth defects in some of the babies.

Whenever a vital, naturally occurring substance such as L-histidine is injected into the body subcutaneously or intramuscularly (alongside heavy metals, live/attenuated viruses, detergents & antibiotic excipients etc), a counter effect inevitably occurs wherein the immune system cannot differentiate between the naturally occurring amino acid in the body from that present in the vaccine; registering all these intruders as a common enemy of toxic debris. The immune system instinctively kicks into overdrive, alerting any available antibodies throughout the body to identify & eliminate deposits of L-histidine it encounters in its path.

The end result, in each case, we're seeing the antithesis of nature's course develop, as the body, stripped of one or more primary components, is now, in essence, at war with itself. What follows is a cascade of unfortunate auto-immune reactions; neurological & neuro-developmental breakdown.

"I am here today because my daughter was harmed by the Gardasil vaccine. My daughter was actually sterilized by the vaccine. I am begging you, do not expand this vaccine until there are answers to the problems that have already arisen. How many children will have to die because this vaccine was a mistake of crazy proportion? How many will be sterilized?"

From another Gardasil victim's mother:

'HPV Gardasil Vaccine Killed Our Daughter: This is our daughter Jessica Ericzon, one day we came home from work and found her dead on the bathroom floor. An honor student, an all star athlete, never a medical condition in her life. When the coroner called and said her heart just stopped, she was dead before she hit the floor and he couldn't tell why, we just couldn't believe it.

The 3 doses required to complete the HPV vaccination regime are so intense, nurses administering the injections are advised to ask patients to lay down during the procedure. In many instances girls have fainted on the spot or gone into sudden seizures.

Think twice. The Gardasil Vaccine is completely unnecessary, and extraordinarily hazardous to her health."

Vaccine Resistance Movement

Young Girl Wheelchair Bound After Merck's Gardasil, Mom Sues

February 23, 2024

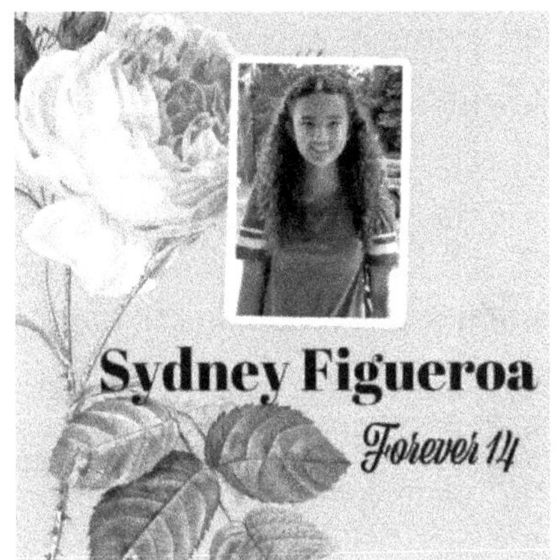


Sydney Figueroa was a happy, healthy, vibrant 11 year old Pennsylvania girl when she received the first dose of Merck's HPV vaccine, Gardasil, on December 6, 2017. She went on and got the second dose of the vaccine when she was 12.

Before the vaccine, Sydney was athletic and very involved in school. She played soccer, was on the track team, and played in the school band. She was a shining star with a bright future.

After the Gardasil shots, Sydney's world fell apart. The young girl developed headaches, brain fog, dizziness, rapid heart rate, exhaustion, leg pain, ringing in the ears, light sensitivity, vision issues, respiratory complications, muscle weakness, inability to walk normally, inability to swallow that ultimately lead to a feeding tube, and excruciating nerve pain.

Sydney was completely left disabled after the vaccine. She was confined to a wheelchair and required full time care. She was diagnosed with Postural Orthostatic Tachycardia Syndrome (POTS), Tourette's Syndrome, and Functional Neurological Disorder.

On June 2, 2021, Sydney died from a pulmonary embolism directly attributable to prolonged immobility because of her autoimmune diseases triggered by Gardasil.

Sydney Figueroa is the latest victim to join Wisner Baum's class action lawsuit against Merck which now has over 150 cases pending.

Sydney's mother Lynne told the attorneys at Wisner Baum, "Gardasil destroyed my daughter's life. She fought for as long as she could but the injuries she suffered, ultimately, killed her. If I knew what I know now, I never would have let Sydney get the shots."

The class action lawsuit also includes Isabella Zuggi, a 10 year old girl who developed a fatal autoimmune disease in the weeks following a single Gardasil shot which caused her death.

http://vaccineresistancemovement.org

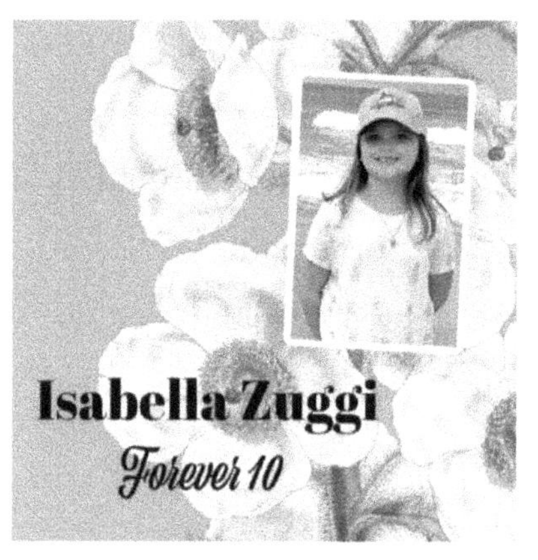


Mother of 10 Year Old Girl Who Developed Fatal Disease After Gardasil Sues Merck

February 22, 2024

I will include the original story along with comments, research and opinions.

"The parents of a North Carolina girl have filed a wrongful death lawsuit after their daughter, Isabella Zuggi, aged 10, developed a fatal autoimmune disease and died 10 weeks after the first dose of Merck's Gardasil vaccine. The child's health declined rapidly after the shot, developing MOG (Myelin oligodendrocyte glycoprotein) antibodies and encephalitis (brain inflammation) where her body attacked the protective myelin coating of her nerves.

Gardasil is marketed as a "prevention" of cervical cancer, by preventing infections with *human papillomavirus*, even though the majority of HPV infections resolve on their own and never develop into cancer. Over 90% of people who are sexually active will be infected with *human papillomavirus* over their lifetime, while very few women will have an undetected, decades-long chronic infection that ever turns into cancer. Death from cervical cancer is rare, representing 0.7% of all cancer deaths.

The majority of cervical cancer deaths in the world occur in developing countries where co-infections with HIV increase one's risk of cervical cancer. Even still, the mortality rate from cervical cancer in Sub-Saharan Africa is still lower than the mortality rate from Merck's Gardasil clinical trial. Read more about *human papillomavirus*.

Isabelle Zuggi's Story

Isabella Zuggi (a twin) was 10 years old when she received the first dose of Merck's Gardasil vaccine, which targets the human papillomavirus, on August 26, 2022.

Two weeks after the shot, Isabella developed headaches, which she never had before. Shortly after this, she had what appeared to be "viral" illnesses. By mid-October, Isabella developed what was thought to be a nastier virus, extreme fatigue, high fever, vomiting, headaches, etc. They went to the doctor, but assumed it was a virus. After this, she appeared to be getting better.

A few days later, Isabella still had the headache so they went to Urgent care, and then Children's Hospital. She was treated for migraines and monitored, and released. She appeared to be getting better.

But a day or so later, Isabella collapsed when she was in the bathroom, covered in sweat and couldn't get up. She was rushed to the hospital.

From that moment on, Isabella could not walk on her own.

In the hospital, she underwent a series of tests, including lumbar punctures, had personality changes, couldn't walk, and lost her ability to speak. Within 48 hours she was on a ventilator, and then on November 5, Isabella Zuggi, died of encephalitis.

Isabella died on November 5, 2022. The cause of death was listed as Acute Encephalitis Associated with Anti-MOG Antibody Production.

Their mother, Kristine, wants people to learn the truth and to not make the same mistake she did. She believes everyone deserves to know the risks of vaccination, and to have proper informed consent.

My heart breaks for their sweet mom. I couldn't imagine what she is going through, knowing she trusted both her physician and the vaccine makers, and now her beautiful daughter is gone. I hope this tragedy saves other lives.

## About MOG Antibody Disease

MOG antibody disease (MOGAD) is a neurological, immune-mediated disorder in which there is inflammation in the optic nerve, spinal cord and/or brain. Myelin oligodendrocyte glycoprotein (MOG) is a protein that is located on the surface of myelin sheaths in the central nervous system.

The diagnosis is confirmed when MOG antibodies in the blood are found in patients who have repeated inflammatory attacks of the central nervous system.

Symptoms of MOG Antibody Disease can vary from patient to patient, and include issues with vision, symptoms association with damage to spinal cord, seizures, paralysis, pain in the eyes, loss of sensation, bladder or bowel problems, confusion, drowsiness or coma.

According to CHOP, which is the hospital associated with Paul Offit:

*"The exact cause of MOGAD is not known. MOG antibody disease affects males and females almost equally and is more prevalent in children than adults."*

Isn't it interesting how so many conditions that could be related to vaccines have causes which are publicly "unknown"?

If it is more prevalent in children than adults, could the CDC pediatric vaccine schedule, which has grown exponentially over the years, be a driver of some or most of the cases of MOG disease? (see links in appendix section)

How can a parent sue a vaccine maker?

The National Childhood Vaccine Act of 1986 prohibits certain failures to warn and design defect claims against manufacturers, but federal law does allow for negligence claims. Plaintiffs who wish to sue a vaccine maker must first file a petition in vaccine injury court, in order to then file a federal negligence claim.

In this case, Gardasil's clinical trial shows many key lines of potential fraud and actively covered up a safety signal of autoimmune disease. Lawsuits fortunately will bring discovery, and we will learn more about just how fraudulent Merck really is.

In Sept. 2022, Merck's lawyers requested that the court limit, discover and provide a speedy process to dismiss claims.

As of February 2, 2023, there are 132 cases in the Gardasil class action lawsuit."

**Feds Sued for Secrets on HPV Vaccine Deaths**

November 2, 2013 This article was posted by TLB Staff HEALTH 4 By: Alyssa Farah.

WASHINGTON – A widely popular HPV vaccine the federal government has recommended for girls and boys as young as 11 has caused thousands of adverse reactions, including seizures, paralysis, blindness, pancreatitis, speech problems, short-term memory loss, Guillain-Barré syndrome and even death.

Now a government watchdog is suing the federal government, demanding it release records related to the vaccine for the sexually transmitted disease human papillomavirus, or HPV.

Judicial Watch announced that it filed a Feb. 14, 2013, Freedom of Information Act lawsuit against the Department of Health and Human Services to obtain those records. The group is seeking records related to the Vaccine Injury Compensation Program, or VICP, a program that compensates patients who have been adversely affected by vaccines. (TLB: see attached Judicial Watch article below)

The HHS website describes the program as a “no-fault alternative to the traditional tort system.”

Judicial Watch wants all records relating to the VICP, any documented injuries or deaths associated with HPV vaccines and all records of compensation paid to the claimants following injury or death allegedly associated with the HPV vaccines.

HHS originally received the FOIA request on Nov. 2, 2012. The department was required by law to respond by Dec. 4. However, as of the date of Judicial Watch’s lawsuit, the agency has failed to provide the documents, indicate when a response is forthcoming or explain why the records should be exempted from disclosure.

The number of successful claims made under the VICP to victims of HPV will provide further information about any dangers of the vaccine, including the number of well-substantiated cases of adverse reactions.

According to the Annals of Medicine: "At present there are no significant data showing that either Gardasil or Cervarix (GlaxoSmithKline) can prevent any type of cervical cancer since the testing period employed was too short to evaluate long-term benefits of HPV vaccination."

"From the very beginning the federal government has attempted to shield the public from the truth about Gardasil," Judicial Watch President Tom Fitton said in a statement. "Despite safety concerns, the vaccine continues to be pushed for both girls and boys.

"For the supposed most transparent administration in history to stonewall on an urgent matter of public health is particularly galling."

In addition to obtaining records from the FDA through the agency's Vaccine Adverse Event Reporting System, which has documented thousands of adverse reactions to Gardasil, Judicial Watch also published a special report in 2008 detailing Gardasil's approval process, side effects, safety concerns and marketing practices.

Dr. Joseph Mercola has noted that the pharmaceutical companies making billions from the vaccines have spent a substantial portion of those revenues on promoting the drugs to doctors, universities, health journals, the Food and Drug Administration and CDC.

Mercola cited other side effects, including:

• *Bell's Palsy and Guillan-Barre syndrome;* • *seizures;* • *cervical dysplasia and cervical cancer;* • *blood clotting and heart problems, including cardiac arrest;* • *miscarriages and fetal abnormalities amongst pregnant women;* • *vaccinated women show an increased number of precancerous lesions caused by strains of HPV other than HPV-16 and HPV-18.*

"It's clear to me that this is another case where the precautionary principle needs to be applied, as currently no one knows exactly whether or not the vaccine will have any measurable effect as far as lowering cervical cancer rates," Mercola said.

"The results will not be fully apparent until a few decades from now, and in the meantime, countless young girls are being harmed, and we still do not know how Gardasil will affect their long-term health, even if they do not experience any acute side effects."

**JW Investigates HPV Injury Compensation Program**

**Documents Obtained by Judicial Watch Reveal 200 Claims Filed with HHS for HPV Vaccine Injuries and Deaths, 49 Compensated**

*Documents Reveal that the National Vaccine Injury Compensation Program (VICP) has Paid Out Nearly $6 million in*

*Claims to Victims of Controversial HPV (human papillomavirus) Vaccine, including Families of Two Dead*

(Washington, DC) – Judicial Watch announced today that it has received documents from the Department of Health and Human Services (HHS) revealing that its National Vaccine Injury Compensation Program (VICP) has awarded $5,877,710 dollars to 49 victims in claims made against the highly controversial HPV (human papillomavirus) vaccines. To date 200 claims have been filed with VICP, with barely half adjudicated.

The documents came in response to a February 28, 2013, Judicial Watch lawsuit against HHS to force the department to comply with a November 1, 2012, Judicial Watch Freedom of Information Act (FOIA) request (*Judicial Watch v. U.S. Department of Health and Human Services* (No. 1:13-cv-00197)). On March 12, 2013, The Health Resources and Services Administration (HRSA), an agency of HHS, provided Judicial Watch with documents revealing the following information:

- Only 49 of the 200 claims filed have been compensated for injury or death caused from the (HPV) vaccine. Of the 49 compensated claims 47 were for injury caused from (HPV) vaccine the additional 2 claims were for death caused due to the vaccine.
- 92 (nearly half) of the total 200 claims filed are still pending. Of those pending claims 87 of the claims against (HPV) vaccine were filed for injury, the remaining 5 claims were filed for death.

- 59 claims have been dismissed outright by VICP. The alleged victims were not compensated for their claims against the HPV vaccine. Of the claims dismissed, 57 were for injuries, 2 were for deaths allegedly caused by the HPV vaccine.
- The amount awarded to the 49 claims compensated totaled 5,877,710.87 dollars. This amounts to approximately $120,000 per claim.

VICP is a Health and Human Services program that compensates patients who have been adversely affected by certain vaccines. The HHS web site **describes the program** as a "no-fault alternative to the traditional tort system," and it covers 16 specific classes of vaccines, **including HPV vaccines** which were added in 2007.

From its inception, the use of HPV (human papillomavirus) vaccines for sexually transmitted diseases has been hotly disputed. According to the *Annals of Medicine*: "At present there are no significant data showing that either Gardasil or Cervarix (GlaxoSmithKline) can prevent any type of cervical cancer since the testing period employed was too short to evaluate long-term benefits of HPV vaccination."

"This new information from the government shows that the serious safety concerns about the use of Gardasil have been well-founded," said Judicial Watch President Tom Fitton. "Public health officials should stop pushing Gardasil on children."

In addition to obtaining records from the FDA through the agency's Vaccine Adverse Event Reporting System (VAERS) which has documented thousands of adverse reactions to Gardasil, Judicial Watch also published a **special report** in 2008 detailing Gardasil's approval process, side effects, safety concerns and marketing practices."

So sad, indeed, are the stories that could have been so easily prevented, and the lives preserved. So many "unknown causes" of death seem to follow a multitude of vaccine injured cases, in denial by the medical establishment.

Gardasil, and the other brand names, for the "protection of HPV" are some of the newer vaccines, more recently created. As we have shown before (and will talk about again later), the very idea of injecting a virus (or any material) to protect against a virus, or any disease (or disease process,) is nonsense. If only people had the proper idea of disease in mind, they would have no motivation to be fear-mongered into taking a substance that is likely to create the very disease it is being touted to prevent. This is a great example of the creation of a vehicle of mass destruction powered by The Germ Theory of Disease (which has become the Viral Theory of Disease).

Every one of the cases of these girls (and now boys) who have experienced loss of function and motor nerve damage, to the lesser problematic dizziness and fainting spells, to the ultimate symptom, of death, was completely unnecessary. It should have never happened! Of course, they have never received affirmation of the success of the vaccine, and they never will. The only hope these victims have is to receive compensation for their loss, but these aren't the sort of losses that can be compensated.

## The Polio Mystery

Before we move on, I do just want to talk about one other vaccine conundrum, which has to do with the rise of polio. The fact that they still give this toxin to children, after it should be well known what truly caused the polio epidemic in the first place, is confounding.

The word, Polio, is a misnomer. It is thought of, and declared so by the medical establishment, as a viral disease, but the history of Polio shows us a different theory for disease than what was thought to be, previously.

According to the history of the word: *Polio* means "gray" in Greek. *Myelitis* means inflammation. Thus the word poliomyelitis means the inflammation of the spinal cord (or gray matter).

According to online sources: "Poliovirus" (and other non-polio viruses) are, supposedly, enteroviruses that spread via the fecal oral route that in 95% of cases is completely asymptomatic, meaning it produces *no symptoms*. A few people will have some mild symptoms, such as flu-like symptoms: fever, fatigue, nausea, stomach pain, etc. Paralysis is a very rare and atypical consequence of a poliovirus infection. Some resources say, it occurs in about 1 in 200 cases of poliovirus infection, or less than 1% of the time." This is the definition you'll most commonly find upon researching the topic.

I must, briefly, point out the fact that the "virus" claimed to be the culprit for this very devastating and possibly life-altering disease, is stated to not produce the same effect in all patients (or people) with whom it is found. In other words, some people who carry this "virus" are perfectly healthy and normal, while others who carry it become paralyzed. Why?? May I ask, are we blaming the paralysis on a virus that, clearly, does NOT consistently deliver certain symptoms?

Infections can result from bacteria in feces, mud and other contaminated matter that enters the system through a cut or injury. This can produce inflammation and cause swelling, pain, fever and other symptoms related to such infections.

The Central Nervous System attack that produced the paralysis (and spinal cord damage) that was the trademark of Polio, was discovered to be genetically hazardous products, such as DDT, and other insecticides being routinely sprayed during the time the "outbreaks" occurred. These products were literally designed to damage the CNS of certain pests. They were supposed to be "harmless to humans" but I guess we know now they weren't. In the 1950s a physician named Dr. Morton S. Biskind testified before congress that polio was a result of central nervous system poison, not a virus. This was a blow to several legislators at the time, who had just awarded Paul Herman Miller the Nobel Prize in Physiology or Medicine in 1948 for his discovery of the High efficiency of DDT as a contact poison against several arthropods. By October of 1945, DDT was being heavily promoted as an agricultural and household pesticide.

Polio was too obvious to miss, for those willing to look. Yet, this information will not be what you'll find upon "googling the subject." They still say that polio is caused by a virus. Well, the fact that they still offer a vaccine for it, means they must. Yet, none of the damage that caused any of the paralysis so devastating to the "polio" victims is something you can vaccinate against or create an immunity to.

It really should make you stop and wonder.

I will tie in some of this to the sections on SCIENCE and on Disease THEORY, but let's first at least touch on one of the most recent "pandemics" that propelled so many vaccine injections.

# CHAPTER 5

# THE COVID-19 "VIRUS"

The thrust, and desperate cry of the "COVID 19 virus" caused many to feel pressured into allowing a doctor or medical assistant to inject them with toxins and substances they had no idea the impact of. I have heard and witnessed more horror stories in the last few years than I would have wished to hear about in a lifetime. People with nervous system disorders, extreme, unexplained, and debilitating pain, loss of use of their limbs, loss of their infant child, sudden onset diabetes, other organ failure, cancer, and a myriad of other lesser issues, like headaches, foggy-mindedness, difficulty breathing, GI distress etc. The varying degrees of sudden onset issues are about as diverse as one might imagine, and did not affect everyone equally, making it easier for the medical establishment to blame them all on coincidence.

Some of the more sudden and extreme, that are particularly hard to call coincidence, and which happened on not just a large, but very personal scale, were among athletes who seemed to be in their prime, physically fit and loving life who became bed-ridden due to loss of mobility, became overwhelmed with excruciating nerve pain to the point they could not sleep and barely function, and also many who mysteriously died within days, weeks or months of receiving a vaccine, or round of vaccines. I wish I had kept a diary, at the time, of the stories I heard. There are many I cannot find anymore, and some I cannot even remember the names of the victims. I'm not sure I wanted to remember, at the time. But these are, again, stories that must not be forgotten!

Many, many stories are impossible to deny the correlation, as some of them reported instant swelling and pain at the injection site that spread to the rest of their body and worsened until they either lost their life or the quality of it. Yet, you won't find any of these stories on mainstream searches, and many of them streamed only for a short time before being removed due to "fact-checkers" or other labels like "false information" or "offensive content" etc. Others just seem to fade into the background.

## The sudden Death of Athletes.

In 2020, there were multiple deaths related to the COVID Vaccines, yet every excuse you could come up with was made for why people were collapsing and dying. An article I found online boldly proclaims, "Vaccine Theory About Footballers Collapsing Debunked." The story about Christian Erikson, who collapsed suddenly on the field, June 12, 2021. His heart stopped for 5 minutes. His story is one of the most inspirational comebacks of football (soccer) history. He was one of the many who collapsed suddenly after receiving the pushed, mandatory COVID vaccines. The claim on the website news.com.au is that his cause for collapse is unknown, even though, also included in the article is the undisputable fact (expressed in a video pop up) that Pericarditis is a "very rare" side effect of vaccines. In this same video, telegraph reporter Georgia Clark is being interviewed on this topic, because she was a victim whose Pericarditis was obviously linked to the Vaccine, yet she is shown as quoting that "they can have side effects but they're rare." In the same video, she encourages people to still get the COVID Vaccine because the "COVID-19 virus is more deadly overall." Myocarditis is inflammation of the heart muscle (while pericarditis is inflammation of the tissue, or sac that surrounds the heart) and this is a direct effect of the ingredients of the Vaccine. I found it interesting, and appalling, that the CDC director, Yvonne Maldonado was introduced (near the end of the same video) as the one to listen to the advice of, and she urged people to get their vaccine reminding them of the "dangers of COVID that is killing people every day."

It is sad, so many still don't know by now that **Vaccine Damage is Not Rare**, and that **a COVID virus was Not causing the high toll of death rates.**

Let us look at another story, right around the same time: Story by Olivia Kelleher from the *Irish Mirror*

**20:00, 24 SEP 2024**

"The family of a talented footballer who died five days after he got a COVID vaccine have told an inquest that they just want to establish the truth about what happened to him.

Roy Butler, of O'Reilly Road in Waterford, died on August 17, 2021, at Cork University Hospital (CUH), having been hospitalized the previous day. He was brought to the hospital by ambulance after suffering from convulsions, jerking and stroke-like symptoms.

Cork Coroner's Court was told that the sports-loving Villa Football Club player loved life and was respectful, kind and fun loving. His father Martin said that Roy was apprehensive about getting the Covid jab. The young man received the Janssen (Johnson and Johnson) one-jab vaccine on August 12, 2021.

Mr. Butler said his son, who was a "very healthy 23-year-old", only got the vaccine because he wanted to go to Dubai with his friends. He went to a pharmacy for the vaccine and when he returned, Mr. Butler said that Roy "looked shook." He recalled that Roy went to work at Bausch and Lomb as usual in the following days. Roy told his father that he had had a "bad night" on the Saturday night. However, diligent as ever, the conscientious young man opted to go to work on Sunday. On

August 16, Roy had a few days off, having completed his run of shift work. Roy decided to go to a gym at about 2.30pm but was home within a very short period of time. Mr. Butler said that Roy complained of feeling unwell. Mr. Butler indicated that it was very unusual for Roy to be sick. The upbeat young man wasn't a person for "complaining about a headache," he said. He said his wife Angela got Roy to bed. Within ten minutes, Roy was texting her to come up the stairs. The concerned father then detailed the shocking scenes he encountered in his son's room.

"Roy's eyes were closed even though he was getting sick and I kept talking to him to get him to respond. Roy was getting sick as he lay on the bed and in convulsions. Angela rang 999 [911] and got through to the ambulance. It was maybe half an hour before they arrived. Roy did not improve this time. He was just jerking... convulsions from side to side."

The paramedics called a second ambulance as they needed sufficient manpower to lift the very ill young man out of the house. Mr. Butler said his son's condition continued to go downhill. "They (the paramedic) told me to keep talking to him and I held his hand. Roy was unresponsive. The second ambulance arrived. We were not allowed in the ambulance. So we followed on."

Mr. Butler said that Roy was taken to University Hospital Waterford for treatment. A family liaison gave them regular updates. He said that the family were informed that "they had never seen anything like this before." A decision was made to transfer Roy to Cork University Hospital (CUH) at 8pm on August 16, 2021.

Mr. Butler said that while they were on the way to Cork, they got a call from a neurosurgeon who informed them that their youngest son only had a two per cent chance of survival. "I asked him to do his best. Twenty minutes later, we got a call from the surgeon again. He said things had gotten worse and he said there was only a one per cent chance now."

The following day, the Butler family were informed that, despite the best efforts of medics, nothing could be done for Roy. Mr. Butler said that it was important to him that the "truth be told" as to what occurred to his son. A decision was made to take Roy off life support and he passed away within a matter of minutes.

Mr. Butler said that his son "didn't look himself" when he came home from having the vaccine. He indicated that Roy was passionate about sport. "He never missed a training session. He would do anything to go. He was captain of every team he played for. He was always fit and healthy. He was strong and tall. He was always training. We got on absolutely fantastically," he said.

Mr. Butler said that "walking out as a captain under the tunnel" was always something Roy wanted to do and he achieved that in life. The family live across the road from Waterford United and Roy always wanted to play with the team. Luckily, he realized his dream.

Meanwhile, Angela Butler stated that Roy was a "perfectly healthy young man" prior to taking the vaccine._She stated that she just "wanted the truth'' about what happened to her younger son. Although, he had asthma as a youngster, his mother said that it had no bearing on his health and that he had "used an inhaler twice in his life."

She said that when Roy went to the gym on August 16 he returned in a very short period of time. "He came back after thirty minutes. I knew something was wrong. He was very pale. He said his heart was banging (out of his chest)."

Mrs. Butler said that "Roy was perfectly healthy and happy." "He was perfect and then he got the injection and he wasn't perfect." She stated that Roy "loved living and did a lot in his short life." "We miss him every second of every day," she said, adding that "her baby boy" Roy was "always happy and positive."

Aaron Butler, the older brother of the deceased, said that although there was a seven-year age gap between them, he always enjoyed a fantastic relationship with his brother. He described Roy as "the complete package."

He said that two days after Roy got the vaccine, he texted him and said he had headaches, and was sweaty, groggy and had a sore jaw and neck. Roy told Aaron via text: "I'm not dying but I'm not well." Roy also texted six of his friends in the days after he got the vaccine saying that he felt unwell.

Paramedic Brian Jackman said that Roy was "unresponsive" when the ambulance crew arrived onsite at around 5pm on August 16, 2021. He stated that Roy was "showing signs of having a stroke." He stated that it was an "emergency situation" and that Roy was "seizing" when they arrived at the hospital in Waterford."

Five days after. It's pretty hard to call it coincidence when there is literally no other explanation and The COVID Vaccines were Known to have side effects. Very serious side effects, and NOT at all RARE.

Before the 2022 FIFA world cup kicked off there was an Instagram post causing more than a bit of a stir, claiming *108 FIFA regular players died in the six months prior.* Many of these professional soccer players had just received their 2nd dose of the COVID-19 Vaccine. The original post, on December 6th, 2021, was flagged as part of FB efforts to "combat False News". Indeed, every time someone mentioned the COVID Vaccines in a negative light, the post was flagged and usually taken down. I have, personally, watched stories appear, often heart-wrenching, and then get removed, days, and sometimes just hours later. The original post was on an Israeli news sight. 108 athletes, all from heart-related illnesses, yet they try to debunk and explain it all away and say there were "other" reasons.

A more thorough article, hopefully, you can still find online, but I am recording here, almost in full: From: BRUCE

FOSTER To: DPBH State BOH Subject: **At least 69 athletes collapse in one month, many dead**

Date: Monday, December 6, 2021, 9:43:58 PM

The reports of athletes who suddenly collapsed have been increasing noticeably lately. Heart problems such as heart inflammation are often the cause – one of the known life-threatening side effects of Covid vaccines, which even the manufacturers themselves warn against.

The current phenomenon is also evident if you simply look on Wikipedia at the list of footballers who have collapsed and died. The year 2021 stands out with 13 entries so far. In no other year mentioned have more footballers died during a game. And this list goes back to the year 1889. So, it really is a historical event. The mainstream media is curiously uninterested in this major global story.

The German online outlet *Wochenblick* compiled a referenced list of the cardiac incidents in October while another online outlet *Granite Grok* published a new list of sportsmen collapsing on the field. Other outlets also listed these incidents, with some cases overlapping. But these do not include Filipino professional basketball star Roider Cabrera who on Wednesday collapsed during tournament play in Pasig City. The Tribune from the Philippines reported he had a cardiac arrest. Roider Cabrera later lost consciousness inside the locker room before he was immediately rushed to hospital where he was diagnosed with fatal arrhythmia according to a local news. Many top athletes from both Europe and the US have reported serious side effects after a Covid jab. For French professional tennis player Jérémy Chardy, it has meant the end of his career. Chardy, formerly ranked 73 in the world, said he has been unable to train and play. "Since I got my vaccine [between the Olympics and the US Open], I have a problem, I have a series of problems. As a result, I can't train, I can't play." Icelandic professional footballer Emil Pálsson (28) collapsed in the game between his club Sogndal IL and Stjørdals/Blink. As reported by *German daily Bild, Pálsson* collapsed during the game, according to the Norwegian broadcaster NRK and the newspaper Verdens Gang. According to his club, he suffered cardiac arrest and had to be resuscitated. This week, on November 24, in the middle of the second half of the game between Reading FC and Sheffield United, Sheffield player John Fleck (30) suddenly collapsed on the field due to a cardiac incident and had to be rushed to hospital. Soccer star from Sheriff Tiraspol Adama Traore went down while holding his chest during the Champions League game against Real Madrid on Wednesday night. In Montana, a Park City High School football player Jedd Hoffman, passed away this month, almost one week after collapsing on the field during practice. These are cases not yet listed in the ongoing carnage that the jabs have unleashed. In October cardiac and circulatory events on the sports field went through the roof.

Below is a shockingly long list of athletes who collapsed last month from heart problems or circulatory disorders such as strokes. Unfortunately, some of these incidents were fatal for the often very young athletes. The numbers are alarming, especially in view of mandatory Covid shots.

(1) At the encounter between PGS E Bosico and Romeo Menti (Allerona Scalo) in Umbria/Italy on October 2, 2021 , a "young player" from the visiting team collapses without any external influence and is transported to the hospital.

(2) Martin Lefèvre (16) from FC Agneaux collapses without any previous illnesses with a stroke during the game against FC Saint-Lô Manche on October 2, 2021. He is paralyzed on one side and has no ability to speak.

(3) Niels de Wolf, 27, from the Belgian football club White Star Sombeke, suffered a cardiac arrest immediately after the game against Verrebroek on October 3, 2021, was resuscitated with a defibrillator, but died in hospital on October 6, 2021 .

(4) Arcisate, Province of Varese, Italy: The amateur match between Valceresio and Tradate (Prima Categoria, Girone A) is canceled after 20 minutes after the referee suffers a medical emergency . Message from October 3, 2021.

(5) Timucin Sen from Germania Großkrotzenburg will be substituted on October 3, 2021 in the game against Spvgg. Oberrad. He collapsed after ten minutes into the game and was taken to a clinic in Gelnhausen.

(6) On October 3, 2021, referee Öner Calik, in his mid-30s, canceled the game between VfB Waltrop II and Vinnum II due to his own health problems and was taken to the hospital by the emergency doctor.

(7) On October 4 , 2021, a person in charge of SV SW Frömern collapsed on the field before the game against Kamener SC.

(8) Cleveland, Ohio, USA: Elias Abou Nassif (44) suffers cardiac arrest in the gym and can be saved by using a defibrillator. Message from October 5, 2021

(9) Lecco (Italy), October 7, 2021: 17-year-old athlete from Colverde collapses during training with cardiac arrest. Defibrillator insert. He is now fighting for his life in the intensive care unit at Lecco Hospital.

(10) AH player (49) from SC Massay in France suffers a fatal heart attack during a game on October 8, 2021.

(11) The golf caddy Alberto Olguín from Mexico collapses dead on the ninth hole of the tournament in Nuevo Vallarta (Mexico). Message from October 9, 2021.

(12) England: In the League One game between Ipswich Town and Shrewsbury on October 9, 2021, Shrewsbury professional striker Ryan Bowman (29) has to be taken off the field after a good half hour of play with extreme cardiac arrhythmias and a pulse of 250 and treated with a defibrillator.

(13) Pompeo Tretola, an 18-year-old soccer player from FC Matese, collapses during the game against Vastese Calcio on 10.10.2021 without any warning signs. He is later transported to the hospital.

(14) Normandy, France: After warming up before the match between Saint-James and Avranches on 10 October 2021, 40-year-old player from Saint-James suffers a heart attack and is saved by a fire-medic on the team of Avranches.

(15) 59-year-old long-distance runner from Biella dies of heart failure in a race in northern Italy. Message from 10/10/2021.

(16) In the match between Wacker Mecklenbeck and Fortuna Freudenberg in the Women's Westphalia League on October 10, 2021, a player collapsed without any opposing influence and was transported to the Münster University Hospital.

(17) Argentina: Mayor Guillermo Mercado (50) died of cardiac arrest after participating in the long-distance run "Aventura de Cerezal" . Message from 10/11/2021.

(18) At the Boston Marathon on October 11, 2021, marathon star Megan Roth collapsed after eight miles of racing with cardiac arrest. She can be saved and is waiting for a defibrillator to be implanted.

(19) NBA player Brandon Godwin of the Atlanta Hawks explains that the Covid vaccination had caused severe side effects for him, which would mean that he not only had to end the season, but possibly his entire career. Message from October 12, 2021.

(20) Le Havre, France: A 27-year-old policeman suffers a fatal heart attack while jogging. News from October 12, 2021. (

(21) Ferran Duran, player from the 4 Catalan League (27), suffered cardiac arrest five times during a game on October 12, 2021 and miraculously survived.

(22) France: The player Christophe Da Silva of Saint Avé collapses with cardiac arrest in the AH Cup match between the Locqueltas footballers and Saint Avé . Message from 10/13/2021

(23) Ensenada, Mexico: The 16-year-old student Héctor Manuel Mendoza dies of a "fulminant heart attack" while training in a sports club . Message from 10/13/2021.

(24) Brazil: Atletico Goianiense 's youth footballer Fellipe de Jesus Moreira suffers a heart attack in the training center and later another heart attack in the emergency room. Now he is fighting for his life in the intensive care unit. News from October 14, 2021.

(25) The next referee who breaks down and dies during a game : happened at the Kreisliga B game between SC Daisbach and FSV Taunusstein in Aarbergen on the evening of October 14, 2021 .

(26) The professional cyclist and multiple Italian time trial champion Gianni Moscon (27) is about to have a catheter ablation due to cardiac arrhythmia. News from October 14, 2021.

(27) Joe Plant from Whitby (Yorkshire, England) suffers in 2021 at a race walking competition of all the British Heart Foundation a cardiac arrest, at 14:10, he himself reported.

(28) Lars Schneider, trainer of TV Braach, retires due to lack of strength after he collapsed with cardiac arrhythmias during the game of the district league A Hersfeld / Rotenburg against SG NentershausenWeißenhasel-Solz in Solz and had to be transported to the clinic. Message from 10/14/2021.

(29) Treviso, Italy: 53-year-old AH player suffers a heart attack while training on October 14, 2021 . He could be kept alive by fellow players.

(30) Australia: 14-year-old student Ava Azzopardi suffers cardiac arrest during the game between Runaway Bay and Magic United at Surfers Paradise Apollo Soccer Club. She is resuscitated by nine rescue workers, put into an artificial coma and is now fighting for her life in the hospital. News from October 15, 2021.

(31) At the handball 3G Bundesliga game in Wuppertal between Bergisches HC and HSG Wetzlar on October 16 , 2021 , a spectator with cardiac arrest collapsed not only during the game (this led to the game being abandoned); after the game, a second spectator also suffered a cardiac arrest .

(32) A 16-year-old boy from Idaho collapses when lifting weights with cardiac arrest. He wakes up after two days in a coma, but is

"extremely confused" and has no short-term memory. News from October 16, 2021.

(33) Camposampiero, Province of Padua, Italy: The 37-year-old doctor Filippo Morando dies while jogging. The ambulance flown in by helicopter can no longer do anything as it is too late. Message from 10/17/2021.

(34) The Premier League game between Newcastle United and Tottenham FC on October 17, 2021 was suspended due to a medical emergency in the stands.

(35) Haitem Jabeur Fathallah, 32, a Fortitudo Messina basketball player, suffers cardiac arrest during the game and dies in hospital. Message from 10/17/2021.

(36) Blumenau, Brazil: Former FC Brusque soccer player from the Brazilian second division, Adans Joao Santos Alencar (38) , suffers a fatal cardiac arrest in a footvolley tournament. Message from 10/17/2021.

(37) Lombardy, Italy: A 40-year-old cyclist stops because of "medical emergency" on , falls to the ground, is transported to the hospital by rescue helicopter Rho. Message from 10/17/2021.

(38) Waseem Aslam of Bradford (England) interrupts a game of football suffering from a cardiac arrest. He could be saved by friends. Message from October 18, 2021.

(39) A 26-year-old runner collapses from cardiac arrest in the Detroit Free Press Marathon . Two police officers rescue him with chest compressions. After that he was treated in the hospital. Message from October 19, 2021.

(40) Cardiac arrhythmias force soccer star Sabrina Soravilla to end her career on October 19 , 2021 after 68 international matches for Uruguay.

(41) Real Murcia's Antonio López had to retire at the age of 32 due to a heart disease . Message from October 19, 2021.

(42) A 41-year-old amateur soccer player in Brazil dies of cardiac arrest in a game. It happened on October 19, 2021 in Nao-me-toque (Rio Grande do Sul).

(43) Henry, a teenager from Halifax, England, is recognized for saving the life of his 56-year-old father after a cardiac arrest while jogging in March. Message from October 20, 2021.

(44) At the first division match between Osasuna and Granada in Pamplona on October 22, 2021, a home team fan suffers cardiac arrest and dies in hospital.

(45) Dieppe, France: A jogger collapses while running with cardiac arrest. He is rescued by two police officers on the patrol. Message from 10/22/2021.

(46) Acerra (Italy): Remigio Gova. A basketball referee and nurse, in Italy inevitably "vaccinated" against Covid, at only 30 years of age "died in his sleep". Message from October 23, 2021.

(47) A double medical emergency at an English stadium on 10/23/2021 during the Championship League game between West Brom and Bristol City. Defibrillator used; the game had to be postponed twice.

(48) Belgian soccer player (37) suffered cardiac arrest in the locker room after his club's match on October 24$^{th}$, 2021, was reanimated but died in hospital.

(49) France: 43-year-old US Montgascon goalkeeper dies of cardiac arrest at half-time. Happened on October 24, 2021 at the La Bâtie-Montgascon stadium.

(50) A 53-year-old suffers a triple cardiac arrest in Bilbao half-marathon and passes away as a result. Message from October 24, 2021.

(51) Tevita Brice, 28, of Montclair Rugby Football Club, US, collapsed on the pitch with a heart attack. In critical condition. Message from 10/25/2021.

(52) Fatal cardiac arrest at a mountain running event in the Italian Alps on October 24, 2021. The victim is Bruno Taffarel (56) from Cordenons.

(53) A cardiac arrest of a player overshadowed the top game of the A2 Dortmund regional soccer league. The player from SG Gahmen was hospitalized on 10/24/2021. The affected team had played against Eving Selimiye Spor.

(54) Nocera Umbra, Italy: Sports teacher and soccer coach Mario Mingarelli suffered fatal cardiac arrest during his team's game on October 24, 2021 at the age of 69 .

(55) The amateur match between Frugesport (Ravenna) and Vaccolino (Prima Categoria, Girone F) is canceled after 32 minutes because the "young" referee suffers a medical emergency . Message from 10/26/2021.

(56) 17-year-old Elly Böttcher from Rostocker FC collapsed unconscious during the away game in Hohen Neuendorf of the Frauen Regionalliga Nordost on October 24, 2021 without any interference and was transported to the hospital. The game was stopped after the incident.

(57) A 20-year-old Italian collapses when skateboarding with a cardiac arrest and is now fighting for his life in the hospital in Verona, where he was transported by helicopter. News from October 25, 2021.

(58) A fan of the Belgian second division team from Lier collapsed on October 27, 2021 in the stadium with heart problems and died in hospital.

(59) On the same day (27.10.2021) also in Belgium, the cup match against Dender of Eupen: A fan collapses with cardiac arrest and must be revived.

(60) Sassuolo, Italy: A 53-year-old mountain biker suffers fatal cardiac arrest on an off-road tour. Message from 10/27/2021.

(61) England: A fan collapses after the Cup game Stoke City against Brentford on October 27, 2021 in front of the stadium with cardiac arrest and dies.

(62) A player from Blau-Weiß Linz from Ghana (26) collapses during his club's home game against Hartberg and is transported to the hospital. Happened on October 27, 2021 at the round of 16 for the ÖFB-Pokal. He is diagnosed with a congenital heart rhythm disorder and was helped with a defibrillator.

(63) Pakistan: The 30-year-old player Muhammad Islam from FC Raziq Chaman suffers a heart attack in the middle of the game against Millat Club and dies. Message from 10/28/2021.

(64) The Swedish-Iraqi player Aimar Sher from the Italian first division club Spezia Calcio collapses during training and is transported to the hospital. Message from 10/28/2021.

(65) Pennsylvania, USA: A 12-year-old student at Chartiers Valley Middle School collapses while playing basketball in physical education class without help and dies. Message from 10/28/2021.

(66) Barcelona star Sergio Aguero (33) suddenly gets breathless during the league game against Deportivo Alaves, grabs his chest and collapses. The Argentine national team player must now take a

break of at least three months. A few months ago he was suffering from a severe Corona infection. Notification from 10/30/2021

(67) During the ICE ice hockey league game, Boris Sadecky (24) from the Bratislava Capitals collapses on the ice without any outside interference. He dies five days later. It later emerges that he suffered from "mild myocarditis" on match day. Message from 10/30/2021

(68) The student and soccer coach for the La Salle High School team in Pennsylvania, USA Blake Barklage died after a heart attack over the weekend. Message from 11/1/2021.

(69) Argentina: The soccer player Ronald Biglione dies after the 2nd vaccination due to thrombosis – a well known side effect of the vaccinations against which the manufacturers themselves warned about. He was treated in Cordoba hospital for two weeks. Message from November 5, 2021. B. Foster

A ridiculous number of athletes from all over the world, did NOT all simultaneously collapse as a coincidence! Yet, the media is shockingly uninterested in covering these stories. Oh, yes, because they were too busy trying to maintain their "terrifying" Corona virus narrative. Yes, it was a terrifying time, indeed, but it wasn't a virus that was causing hordes of damage (unless that's what you want to call the poison in the vaccines).

This is only ONE CATEGORY of people who were adversely affected from the COVID vaccine. One that was particularly hard to ignore. The categories of types of people affected are far broader and touch every people group in some way, but many of their experiences are easier to chalk up to "coincidence" or write off as due to a "virus" or other health issue.

Just one, real story of someone reacting to a COVID Vaccine

This story was also taken, and should be able to be found on the Circle of Mammas website.

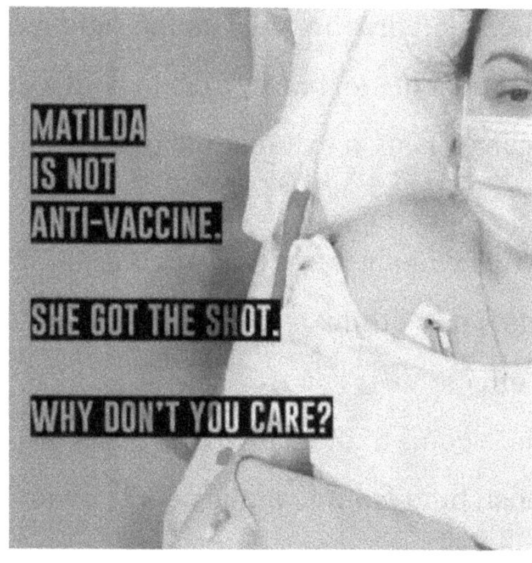


September 19, 2021

*Shared from Matilda:*

"Get the vaccine they say.. Lockdown over..

What the news doesn't tell you is how aggressive the side effects are. Yesterday, I lost control of my body, I could hardly lift up my arms. My eyes would ache to open. To get one word out of my mouth was painful, my tongue struggled to allow sound from my swollen and red throat.

My chest felt pressure, then aches which turned into sharp pains. My heart slowed down making each and every breath harder and harder. Rashes on my chest were sore and red.

I was rushed to hospital last night, to be taken into the emergency room, to be sat down on my own with no one to help. It wasn't until I had to verbally explain I had flu symptoms that they put me in a wheelchair and took me through to be triaged. It was a mess, because I couldn't verbalize what was going on.

I then went straight to bed; my heart rate was incredibly low 84/49. Hooked up and poked and prodded, two nurses and a doctor had to slap my veins to try to get one to do blood tests. This took three attempts in my left arm and two on the right arm. Two drip bags later I started to come to, barely able to hold a cup of water to drink, I have never felt such exhaustion, pain and heaviness.

They don't tell you this when you get the vaccine, and they do not put this on the tv ads. I don't think anyone is prepared for the possible extreme side effects.

I am aware that this is going to open the flood gates of social media hell on this post, but I want to make people aware of what can happen. And for those who push vaccines, or people who are against. Be aware that this is real life, not sugar coated. This is our health and well being at risk.. scary stuff!"

Matilda's "DISCLAIMER** My post is spoken from my emotion and my own experience, which should spread awareness to look after your bodies and do what is right for you!

In no way am I here to sway anyone's opinion. Your body, YOUR CHOICE 💗"

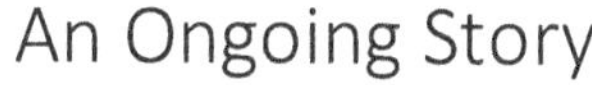


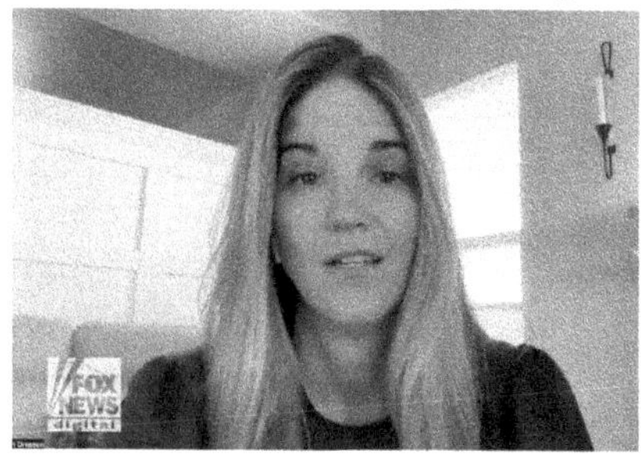


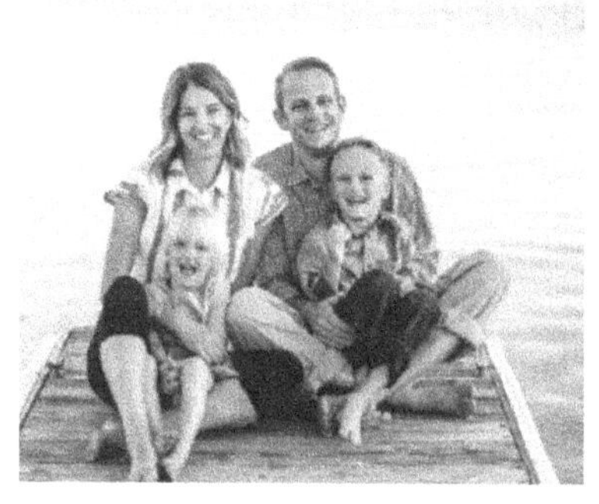

The story of Brianne Dressen, who lost her quality of life, and remains in constant, extreme, debilitating pain after receiving the COVID jab, is truly heart-breaking. She was in perfect health and climbing mountains and teaching before she volunteered to take part in a vaccine trial. She's now been diagnosed with post-vaccine neuropathy, dysautonomia and POTS.

She is attempting to sue the pharmaceutical co. AstraZeneca after they offered her a less than $1,300 payout.

You can view her story on several different platforms through various interviews. A few are currently on YouTube, at the time of writing this.(See Appendix) Her story is profound, as she went from being totally on board with doing everything she could to encourage people to do their part in taking the vaccine and joining together as a community to fight the present pandemic, in line with the narrative being pushed at that time, to now standing, and speaking against the vaccines, because she has, since, learned the truth.

Brianne's story is ongoing, and she still fights for those who are not being heard... (Please check out her story and watch some of the more recent interviews online: Links in the Appendix Section)

The number of people who were negatively effected by the COVID vaccines is not even recordable. The effects still continue to harm and even those who were not vaccinated were, and continue to be, affected due to the mRNA shedding, we are now discovering. (more on this later)

## "Tip of the Iceberg" studies

An article in Lancet Regional Health EU titled: *"The epidemiological relevance of the COVID-19-vaccinated population is increasing"* has important aggregated data on the significance of the vaccinated as sources for transmission of SARS-CoV-2 (1). The article highlights that high COVID-19 vaccination rates have not reduced transmission of SARS-CoV-2 in populations by reducing the number of possible sources for transmission and thereby reduced the burden of COVID-19 disease. Recent data indicates that the epidemiological relevance of COVID-19 vaccinated individuals as a source of transmission is increasing, as there are fewer unvaccinated and more people are naturally immune.

## Vaccine Shedding?

Another paper out of the UK shows that fully vaccinated individuals with breakthrough infections have peak viral loads similar to the unvaccinated, and that fully vaccinated individuals can efficiently transmit infection in household settings. The authors conclude that host–virus interactions early in infection may shape the entire viral trajectory.

In this study, the secondary attack rates among household contacts exposed to fully vaccinated index cases was similar to household contacts exposed to unvaccinated index cases (25% for vaccinated vs 23% for unvaccinated). 12 of 31 infections in fully vaccinated household contacts (39%) arose from fully vaccinated epidemiologically linked index cases. Peak viral load did not differ by vaccination status or variant type

(2). In yet another report by the Robert Koch Institute, it was shown that In Germany, the rate of symptomatic COVID-19 cases among the fully vaccinated ("breakthrough infections", reported weekly since 21, July 2021) was 16.9% at that time among patients of 60 years and older. This proportion has increased weekly and was 58.9% on October 27, 2021. This provides clear evidence of the increasing relevance of the fully vaccinated as a possible source of transmission (3). In the UK, a similar situation shows among citizens of 60 years or older, the fully vaccinated accounted for 89.7% of the SARS-CoV-2 cases versus 3.4% among the unvaccinated (4). A report out of Israel reports a nosocomial outbreak involving 16 healthcare workers, 23 exposed patients and two family members. The source was a fully vaccinated COVID-19 patient. The vaccination rate was 96.2% among all 248 exposed individuals (151 healthcare workers and 97 patients). Out of the 248 people, fourteen fully vaccinated patients became severely ill or died, and two unvaccinated patients developed mild disease (5). The US Centers for Disease Control and Prevention (CDC) identifies four of the top five counties with the highest percentage of fully vaccinated population (99.9– 84.3%) as "high" transmission counties (6). The initial analysis of the Omicron variant is that it is less virulent and more transmissible. Early data also suggests that the current vaccines, developed against the Alpha strain of COVID, are not that useful in stopping transmission. Data also suggests that break-through cases of fully vaccinated individuals are going to be the norm with the Omicron variant. The data above should make decision makers question their assumptions that the vaccinated can be excluded as a source of transmission. "It appears to be grossly negligent to ignore the vaccinated population as a possible and relevant source of transmission when deciding about public health control measures."

There are reasons that the COVID vaccine "sheds" and it is due to the mRNA particles that signal the body to create "spike protein" by the body and this "informational pattern" can be passed on to others: even those who have not been vaccinated."

Note: For More Info, ***Please read the article posted at the end of this book in the Appendix on Vaccine shedding for some of the latest data and research on the matter.***

It should seem beyond negligent, to deny all correlation of death and cardiac malfunction to vaccine administration. Again, this is far from all correlated and causative events related to vaccine damage, on this issue. But these are some of the stories that "made it out" to the surface and received media attention, because it is a little impossible to ignore hundreds, or thousands of famous athletes falling over or passing out on the field. Athletes are one of nature's wonders, who portray the glorious way our creator made our body and its ability to shine when pushed to the limits. It should be no wonder that, when compromised by an inward attack, of poisoning and hardening, the heart gives under the strain and can no longer supply the body. This was not isolated to famous athletes. I, personally, and you probably did too, witnessed many instances that young men (and women) collapsed, suddenly. Some recovered. Many did not.

The pastor of our previous church was one of those who left us so very suddenly. He and his wife were very physically active. Their parents were alive. People in their family seemed to live a long time (this would seem to negate any "genetic predispositions"). His loss was a great devastation to hundreds, no thousands, of people.

In our own and some previous communities we had been a part of, I watched several dads, and a few moms suddenly become gravely ill. In 2020, a significant number of individuals experienced respiratory issues. During this time the COVID-19 virus was blamed for them. Looking back now, it seems almost laughable and ironic that COVID ("corona virus disease") was also synonymous with SARS (severe, acute respiratory symptom), a name that they have drastically changed the meaning of, as well as the symptoms. Now, it is pretty much the, cold, flu, fever, chills, headache, sore throat, fatigue, body aches or basically, "I feel like I'm going to die!" and everything in between, Virus. I find it interesting that the first major symptom being experienced affected your breath and the second major stage affected your heart.

## Bad Treatment Protocols?

This may seem like a side note, but the repeated cases that I watched happen over and over again involved treatment plans that seemed to ensure death from the initial symptoms. People were dying because "they couldn't breathe." (this was a symptom that was being compared to the 1918 epidemic, which we'll discuss a bit later) It was strange, and I heard many people saying the problem was not that they could not breathe or even that their O2 stats were too low. It seemed there was a problem of converting the oxygen in the lungs. Perhaps we'll never know for sure, but it certainly seemed conspiratorial, and we all were certainly being bombarded by... something: Informational overload? A reduction in our ability to handle stress? Too much stress? A virus? -Sure, if a "Virus" means: "something screwing with our bodies at the informational level."

Yet, I did not personally know anyone who died because they couldn't breathe who stayed out of the hospitals. Not saying people didn't, only that I saw so many cases of death after hospital treatment. (My husband and I were involved in an area of natural health that allowed us to see a bit more cases than just family and friends.) The prescribed treatment plan involved a procedure that literally paralyzed them (step one was administering a paralytic drug) put them on a respirator (which automated breathing for them) and put them about as close to death as was humanly possible without killing them (which was pretty much a drug induced coma, that was supposed to keep them from needing too much oxygen)... until it killed them. I watched a 35-yr-old father of littles (who was experiencing difficulty breathing) go from perfectly healthy to dead in a little over a week after he was subjected to this protocol. I watched the progression in one day (because it was over a week before I was alerted to the story) in literal tears and sobbing before I even reached the end, because I already knew where it was heading. I'd watched it happen a dozen times before just the previous week.

Can I say just a few words about the problems in logic concerning this protocol? First of all, if you are going to die because your lungs are no longer able to function well enough to oxygenate your body, or because your body is reacting to something that is causing your breathing to shut down, or if the oxygen you are breathing in is not sufficient to oxygenate your body, then the protocol that was being used at that time could not, possibly have saved you. (It makes sense to put someone on oxygen if they're not getting enough of it. Yet this was found over and over not to be the solution and so they instead went into this protocol). On the other hand, if there was some sort of pathogen, bacteria etc. that your body was trying to eliminate so extremely that your need for coughing and expelling it was so great that you couldn't breathe in enough oxygen (due to a buildup of congestion) this was the best way to shut down that entire cellular response and ensure your death from it. I'm not saying this was the reason, especially not in every case, but, whatever the cause, the protocol was successful at killing more lives than saving them. Who decided this was the best protocol to use and why was it being used so profoundly, has yet to be answered but, there was certainly an erroneous protocol taking place during this time that proved bad judgement in hindsight.

I had never looked at the worldwide website of statistics (worldometer) until that year and found it profoundly interesting that the actual numbers of lives that "COVID" was taking was significantly less or very close to the deaths from flu the previous year. I do think it vital to point out that this happened before the rollout of the vaccine. It would seem to me that the normal or natural number of deaths that would have happened during the push of the COVID scare was not at all sufficient to mandate a vaccine. It seems to me, it could have been, that they needed more deaths from this hyped-up, to be feared, "viral disease." I know that sounds scandalous, but it was just too insane not to make one wonder. I would wager that as you are reading this, you may also remember some of these things, and perhaps they left you in wonderment too.

One observation worth noting, is that the 2019 "Epidemic" "mirrored the Influenza epidemic of 1918" (so they say) in several ways, from sudden onset of new and strange physical issues and phenomenon to mask wearing. The word influenza itself was created to try and explain (or just name) the strange influences that no one had an explanation for. People were dropping dead in the streets. They were coughing up blood and turning blue (some described people as black). People could not breathe and were hemorrhaging in their brains. (Or so the stories go.) So many died in such a brief period of time; it was a world-wide terror. Now, I don't actually think the 2019, so called, pandemic, was actually even close to the 1918 tragedy, but during a period of time, newscasters kept comparing what was happening to 1918. I thought it strange at the time, but now I think the whole point was to scare people into submitting to the planned agenda.

Now, the reasons people couldn't get oxygen into their lungs due to the COVID-19 "Virus" is a "mystery", that had very little to do with any typical symptoms of disease, or any "virus." I do believe that the sudden bombardment of frequency waves from recently erected phone towers certainly played a part. If you think that sounds ludicrous you should read the book, *The Invisible Rainbow: A History of Electricity and Life* by Aurther Firstenberg. The very best similarities between the two (time periods) were the number of respiratory issues and the amount of electricity surging through the air (which was unparalleled to any time before that). The book, Invisible Rainbow, speaks of this time period briefly, but profoundly. Huge radio towers had just been installed, particularly in the US Navy, that beamed a continuous flow of radio waves, in 1918. And we had just erected huge 5G phone towers, pulsing a new energy level across the world in 2019. It is also significant that the most notably affected (particularly at the onset), were not the aged or infirm, but the young and healthy, from 18-40 or some say 15-40 years of age. It is also notable that, in 1918, repeated attempts to prove the contagion of the disease failed at every turn. So, while an Influenza Virus was blamed for the calamity in 1918, the statistics simply don't match up. Echoes a bit how the Corona Virus was blamed for 2019, when we have worldometer statistics that show deaths from the supposed virus, in 2019, were even less than flu deaths the previous year. Once vaccines were thrust forward (and attempted to be mandated in every school and business) we see a huge climb in deaths from "COVID." (See Chart)

This could surely be another series of study altogether, and I think I will leave it there and stick to the main purpose of this book. However, I will say that vaccinations, in the early 1900s, seemed to be at a low during this time, along with many diseases, so I'm not going to blame it on that. Respiratory issues: "whooping cough" and pneumonia etc. are the ones that show an all-time high on the charts of the United States Whooping Cough mortality rates. But Whooping Cough is generally a bacterial infection, which wasn't the case in 1918. (so now we have elevated stats of whooping cough that really should've been labeled: respiratory issues). It wasn't too long after this scare, though, that administration of vaccines began to rise.

Significantly, deaths and cases of Corona Virus surged after the greatest push of Vaccination. See the chart from the worldometer, which now contains the disclaimer: "**NOTE:** As of April 13, 2024, the **Coronavirus Tracker is no longer being updated** due to the unfeasibility of providing statistically valid global totals, as **the majority of countries have now stopped reporting**. However, historical data remain accessible. Worldometer delivered the most accurate and timely global statistics to users and institutions around the world at a time when this was extremely challenging. We thank everyone who participated in this extraordinary collaborative effort."

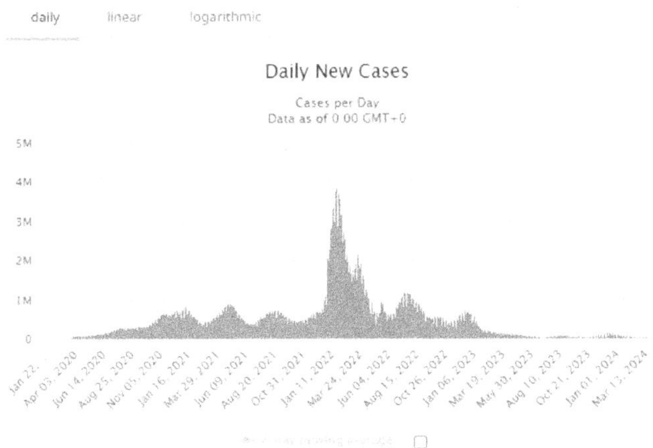


What is crazy is that I don't think I've seen more sickness in the last three years than I have this winter (2024/25), and everyone is calling it COVID. They have this new term now: LONG COVID, to describe prolonged sickness that lasts for weeks, and has severe symptoms. But here we have world-wide "historical data" that makes COVID appear to have vanished after the huge surge of Vaccines. Well, perhaps we need to find a new term to call our bouts of severely prolonged detoxing. It seems to me that people are sicker now than they have been even during previous years. As I said before, there seem to be elements "in the air" or perhaps emanating from the recent toxic overload of "viral information" (like those from vaccine shedding) that just doesn't seem to be going away.

This is far from a comprehensive amount of information on the COVID vaccination, and the effects are still ongoing, the stories far vaster than any here mentioned and the data that I have been able to drudge up (in a timely matter) on the subject is highly insufficient, and there really are no (standard) studies that are informative about the COVID vaccine.

If I am ever able to make a second edition, the section on COVID would certainly be expanded and improved drastically. COVID has left many of us still sifting through the mess trying to make sense of the myriads of voices and data on the matter, and still ongoing repercussions.

Things we do know:

They lied about the Virus.

They lied about the Vaccine.

They gave us terrible advice.

They lost our trust, and now they are trying to re-instate it.

## Other Toxins and Drugs

While there are a few drugs developed over the years, whose side effects (or direct effects) were so devastating they were forcibly removed from the market, we need to realize that many others continued or escaped media attention, or simply caused smaller issues like liver damage, organ damage, or contributed to more chronic conditions, that went unrecognized, or were, instead blamed on VIRUSES.

I am just going to mention a couple here for remembrance' sake.

### Thalidomide

Taken from Wikipedia:

In the late 1950s and early 1960s, the use of thalidomide in 46 countries was prescribed to women who were pregnant or who subsequently became pregnant and consequently resulted in the "biggest anthropogenic medical disaster ever," with more than 10,000 children born with a range of severe deformities, such as phocomelia, as well as thousands of miscarriages.

Thalidomide was introduced in 1953 as a tranquilizer and was later marketed by the German pharmaceutical company Chemie Grünenthal under the trade name Contergan as a medication for anxiety, trouble sleeping, tension, and morning sickness. It was introduced as a sedative and medication for morning sickness without having been tested on pregnant women. While initially deemed to be safe in pregnancy, concerns regarding birth defects were noted in 1961, and the medication was removed from the market in Europe that year.

**Development of thalidomide**

Thalidomide was first developed as a tranquilizer by Swiss pharmaceutical company Ciba in 1953. In 1954, Ciba abandoned the product, and it was acquired by German pharmaceutical company Chemie Grünenthal. The company had been established by Hermann Wirtz Sr, a Nazi Party member, after World War II as a subsidiary of the family's Mäurer & Wirtz company. The company's initial aim was to develop antibiotics for which there was an urgent market need. Wirtz appointed chemist Heinrich Mückter, who had escaped prosecution for war crimes for his experiments on prisoners of Nazi concentration camps, to head the development programme because of his experience researching and producing an anti-typhus vaccine for Nazi Germany. He hired Martin Staemmler, a medical doctor and leading proponent of the Nazi eugenics programme, as head of pathology, as well as Heinz Baumkötter, the chief medical officer at the Sachsenhausen concentration camp, and Otto Ambros, a chemist and Nazi war criminal. Ambros was the chairman of Grünenthal's advisory committee during the development of thalidomide and was a board member when Contergan was being sold.

**Birth defect crisis**

The total number of embryos affected by the use of thalidomide during pregnancy is estimated at more than 10,000, and potentially up to 20,000; of these, approximately 40 percent died at or shortly after the time of birth. Those who survived had limb, eye, urinary tract, and heart defects. Its initial entry into the U.S. market was prevented by Frances Oldham Kelsey at the U.S. Food and Drug Administration (FDA). The birth defects of thalidomide led to the development of greater drug regulation and monitoring in many countries.

The severity and location of the deformities depended on how many days into the pregnancy the mother was before beginning treatment; thalidomide taken on the 20th day of pregnancy caused central brain damage, day 21 would damage the eyes, day 22 the ears and face, day 24 the arms, and leg damage would occur if taken up to day 28. Thalidomide did not damage the fetus if taken after 42 days' gestation.

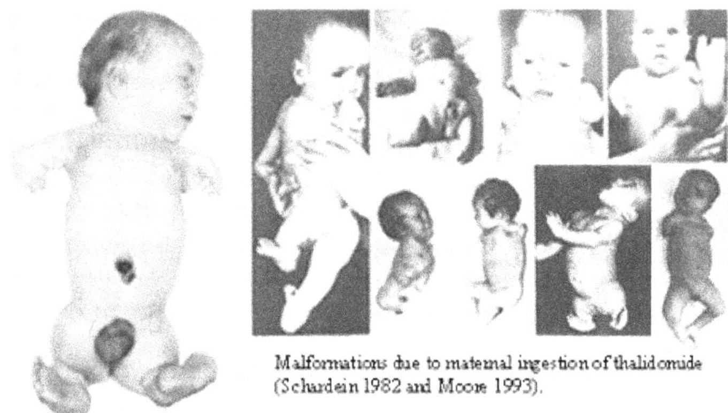

Malformations due to maternal ingestion of thalidomide (Schardein 1982 and Moore 1993).

## Tamiflu

A "flu remedy" produced in 2005, after creating a huge hype about domesticated and game birds dying of an alleged virus. Stories were propelled through the media of people who had become infected or died of the fearful H5N1 "virus". Oseltamivir, or Tamiflu profits reached over a billion dollars in the first 9 mo. of 2006. Then the reports began coming of deaths and psychiatric side effects. The first report was said to be from Japan, that two boys aged 14 and 17 became "disoriented, showed abnormal behavior, and ultimately died. A few days later, reports of the deaths of 12 other children were surfacing in the news. Canadians were reporting cases of hallucinations among Tamiflu users, 84 reports of other side effects and 11 deaths. In the 1990's Tamiflu was known to cause inflammation in the brain (encephalitis). Finally, a comprehensive study evaluation of the Cochrane Collaboration on Tamiflu in 2014, found it "not suitable to prevent the spread of flu or to reduce the occurrence of dangerous complications." Another paper concluded, 3 years earlier that, "taking Tamiflu can lead to sudden deterioration in health and subsequent death."

Never was a true study done to verify the efficacy of Tamiflu, but you can find plenty of Roche -funded studies that, supposedly, prove it works. One of the studies authors, Karl Nicholson, received funding and honorariums from GlaxoSmithKline (who manufactures zanamivir) and Roche, who makes oseltamivir (Tamiflu). British Parliament discovered that 3/4$^{th}$ of the clinical studies in scientific journals, like *The Lancet, The New England Journal of Medicine* and *Journal of the American Medical Association* are all funded by pharmaceutical companies. There are clear conflicts of interest involved and no one to hold these companies accountable for omitting critical questions or negative or unfavorable results, and only publishing what they want the public to see.

This information on Tamiflu was taken from the book *Virus Mania: How the Medical Industry Continually Invents Epidemics, Making Billion-Dollar Profits at Our Expense* by Engelbrecht, Kohnlein, Bailey and Scoglio There is also some great information about the H1N1 Avian Flu, SARS, COVID, Hepatitis, HIV, Polio and other, so called, "viruses", in the Book.

It is filled with history about the REAL CULPRITS of "viral diseases."

I was just reminded about the dangers of ANY FLU "Remedy" offered in hospitals. Just this week (while writing this), I heard a story of a girl (friend of family) who went into the hospital because she "wasn't feeling well" and then her health strangely and rapidly declined after receiving a "flu remedy."

Simply try asking your health advisor/care giver what the ingredients are in the remedy they're offering and how they work. Most can't tell you.

## Drug Induced or Viral?

The book mentioned above, (Virus Mania) has compiled a wonderful history of diseases such as AIDS, Hepatitis and other (so called viral diseases) alongside proof of what was the real, likely culprits.

As just one, quick example: Hepatitis C (HCV) is a disease, purportedly transmitted through blood and blood products. The Cause is attributed to the Hepatitis Virus. It has been discovered that many patients who are experiencing the clinical definition of HPV symptoms often test negative for the antibody. Also, that many who test positive experience no symptoms at all. (Again, why are we blaming a virus for a disease that does not consistently deliver the same symptoms in those who carry said virus?) Other substances as chronic alcoholism, Heroin, as well as the very drug used in the "treatment" of HCV, were seen to produce the liver inflammation associated with the "viral disease" in a far more consistent pattern.

Even emotional factors such as anger, worry or stress conditions that become chronic or extreme seem to be more directly correlated to liver (and other) issues, more than any type of viral (or even bacterial) elements detected in a person.

Perhaps, if we could just take a step back from the mainstream medical narrative for a moment and look at the other surrounding elements, it would reveal the actual cause of each of the diseases that vaccines have been created to exterminate, and if we could remove vaccines altogether along with other toxic medical "treatments," we would certainly see much less disease and death.

In closing this chapter, I want to end with a word of caution and reminder of the consequences that come when recognition becomes misplaced.

It is a morally disturbing historic narrative that gives credit to the destroyer for the improvements we have seen in health and the eradication of disease. If we had been wiser in understanding the realities of health, we would've known we were producing death, not life. Perhaps if we had been humble enough to look to our creator, instead of merely ourselves (or our peers) we would've recognized the conditions that favor life and health, such as cleanliness, better nutrition, proper innovation and gratefulness. For surly it is only by God's Spirit and provision that life and healing come. The great wonderment of such deceptive theology, I believe, lies in the belief that proliferation of disease and death processes could somehow be the answer (but, I suppose that was the great lie from the beginning.) In hindsight, when light is later shed on such eras, the darkness is so evident, in a world that was proclaiming, "Enlightenment" yet, brought the world un-imaginable sorrow.

This is the very reason that we MUST go back into history and dig up the buried realities that contributed to the pain and devastation that we experience in the present. This includes the THEORIES and IDEAS that allowed them in the first place. This is what I want to talk about in the next three chapters.

# CHAPTER 6

# THE SCIENCE

I find it sad, but far too common, that doctors have little knowledge about what they are administering to others. Particularly with vaccines, as all they are told is the hype about them being "safe and effective," neither of which they are.

As a mom who has had to deal with the effects of Iso-immunization (a condition that causes my body to attack the blood cells of my unborn baby, because it is a foreign blood type) I understand a bit about how immunity works. The way the RhoGAM shot, which is designed for Negative blood carriers (moms) of positive blood babies, works may be one of the few good reasons for flooding your system with antibodies, and must be administered within 72 hours of exposure to the foreign (positive) blood type, in hopes that it will be successful at preventing your own body from creating its own antibodies. I can't tell you how many nurses tried to tell me I should get a RhoGAM shot because they hear the phrase, O Negative blood type, and think, that is the automatic protocol. They have no idea how, or why it works, and that in my case (of already having made my own antibodies) there is literally NO POINT in giving me the shot, and all it will accomplish at this point is flooding my system with even more antibodies, which is the opposite of what I need now.

When the ICU practitioners were administering IgG (Immunoglobulin) therapy to my son, to try to bring down his bilirubin levels, they couldn't even answer the question as to what form he was receiving: blood serum (from someone's blood) or a synthetic form. She had no idea what the IgG actually was and later Googled it. But I was grateful that she was humble and gracious about it.

The truth is that many, if not most, practitioners, mean well, and are just trying to do what has been taught or told to them. What is particularly disturbing (and often hurtful) to witness is a doctor who has to be right and clings, stalwartly, to his already established narrative, because he cannot admit to the reality that he could be wrong. Just as in the previous histories I shared in earlier chapters, the "science" (so called) has already been settled. No one (including the general population) is putting vaccines, themselves on trial. The only arguments are whether their "efficacy is worth the risk", or just how protective they are, or which vaccines are more necessary or less so than others. How can we space them out, or how can we make them "safer"? etc. etc. No one is questioning whether the claims of purported antibody "protection" are actually true.

# How do vaccines work??

Let's start, first, with what the vaccine makers, themselves claim.

As an example: According to a vaccine insert for DTap,

Diphtheria

"320 Diphtheria is an acute toxin-mediated disease caused by toxigenic strains of C diphtheriae.

321 Protection against disease is due to the development of neutralizing antibodies to diphtheria toxin.

322 A serum diphtheria antitoxin level of 0.01 IU/mL is the lowest level giving some degree of

323 protection. Antitoxin levels of at least 0.1 IU/mL are generally regarded as protective. (5) Levels

324 of 1.0 IU/mL have been associated with long-term protection. (6)

325 Tetanus

326 Tetanus is an acute disease caused by an extremely potent neurotoxin produced by C tetani.

327 Protection against disease is due to the development of neutralizing antibodies to tetanus toxin. A

328 serum tetanus antitoxin level of at least 0.01 IU/mL, measured by neutralization assay is

329 considered the minimum protective level. (5) (7) A tetanus antitoxin level ≥0.1 IU/mL as

330 measured by the ELISA used in clinical studies of DAPTACEL is considered protective.

331 Pertussis

332 Pertussis (whooping cough) is a respiratory disease caused by B pertussis. This Gram-negative

333 coccobacillus produces a variety of biologically active components, though their role in either the

334 pathogenesis of, or immunity to, pertussis has not been clearly defined."

(then why are we even talking about this one or continuing to give it?!)

There is a lot of circular reasoning behind why particular vaccines work, and what mechanism of action allows them to work. Diphtheria is the name that's been given to a particular "disease," (and blamed on the bacteria we've also given that name) because it manifests certain symptoms that we classify as this particular disease. As stated online:

Symptoms of respiratory diphtheria are:

- Swollen neck lymph nodes (cervical lymphadenopathy)
- Throat is covered by a gray thick membrane
- Feeling of discomfort or illness
- Difficulty swallowing
- Fever
- Sore Throat
- Cough
- Wheezing

- May cause Respiratory failure

Symptoms of cutaneous diphtheria are;

- Ulcers covered by a gray thick membrane
- Redness
- Swelling
- Pain"

It is also stated that, "Diphtheria is a highly contagious, infectious disease caused by a bacterium called Corynebacterium diphtheriae. People with diphtheria have serious breathing and swallowing problems, and they may develop sores on their skin."

This circular reasoning in defining the diseases by the bacteria, whose names we made up along with their treatment protocols, began in earlier history as we have already discussed. Should it not confound us, that we are continuing to do the same thing today?

## Treatments for Diphtheria:

If you have already been diagnosed with diphtheria, what do they prescribe?

As stated on the Web: "Your healthcare provider will prescribe diphtheria antitoxin to stop damage to your organs. They'll also prescribe antibiotics like penicillin or erythromycin, to fight infection.

People with diphtheria are kept in isolation to prevent others from becoming infected. An infected person is no longer contagious around 48 hours after taking antibiotics. When treatment ends, tests will be run again to make sure the bacteria are gone. Once the bacteria are gone, you will get a vaccine to prevent future infections."

Is no one asking why we need to give a vaccine to someone who has just had Diphtheria?? Apparently, the only preventative is not literally having the disease, along with, said Diphtheria bacteria in it, but only the Diphtheria bacteria/toxins in the vaccine matter??

So much of the information and ideas of how disease propagates is inconsistent and even incoherent.

### What exactly is Diphtheria Antitoxin?

They say: "Diphtheria antitoxin (DAT) is a medication made up of antibodies used in the treatment of diphtheria. It is administered through injection into a vein or muscle. Although rare, severe and immediate anaphylaxis is a risk due to its horse serum base. It is no longer recommended for prevention of diphtheria. Diphtheria is a serious disease transmitted through contact with an infected person or carrier."

While they try to make it sound great, in the most basic form, it is antibodies from horse blood and, as already admitted, the results can be devastating!

I have never heard of anyone ever receiving Diphtheria antitoxin, so the only way I could have something to say is to research the topic, but what I have learned about anti-toxin from this study I share in the next chapter.

I don't think I've ever known anyone who ever got Diphtheria (which is rather astounding when I think about it). Although, after looking at the symptoms, I'I think I may have had "Diphtheria" once and just figured it was swollen glands, difficulty breathing and sore throat due to fighting off this bacterial infection I had. The best news was it passed. I never knew it was anything so "serious as Diphtheria" and fully recovered with no issues and no help from a doctor. I'm wondering if it wasn't a good thing that I didn't know it was anything I should've, as they say, "sought medical treatment immediately" for, or let them give me an antitoxin, so my organs didn't shut down. Perhaps, as can be seen in other treatment protocols, the "Anti-toxin" might be the trigger that actually produces the organ failure it's supposed to "treat".

While I've studied natural health for literally decades, I have felt a little sheepish because until researching for this book, I've never even known what Diphtheria (or many of the other diseases that they offer injections for) even was! I'm still not sure I do. (I'm not sure anyone really does for that matter and I think this may be equally true about most, if not all, the other diseases that people are vaccinated for.) Two things I have consistently noticed about the viral diseases we vaccinate for.

1. Few people, even doctors, know much about how to properly or consistently diagnose these diseases because they are supposed to have been eradicated.

2. When people do receive a diagnosis for any of these diseases, they claim it is extremely serious and will likely lead to death.

If these diseases have been eradicated by vaccines (claim) doesn't that mean the symptoms of the disease should also be eradicated? The difficulty, though, is that nearly all the symptoms of these "serious diseases" are just like any other diseases, except for the serious part. Most practitioners and medical information will agree that diphtheria, measles, pertussis etc. start off like flu or a common cold with fever, congestion, sore throat etc. until the disease develops the more serious and specific conditions.

I think it is also significant to keep in mind that the names of the bacteria and viruses that, supposedly, cause the diseases they are named for, were created (defined) during an era that was unable to recognize or isolate any of them. In fact, we still have not isolated many (if not most or any) of the entities, supposedly, responsible.

Also, the entities that we ARE able to identify as being present in the body have been proven NOT to correlate consistently with the disease symptoms. Many who have been shown to have specific viruses (like Hep. B virus or Influenza etc.) are completely "asymptomatic" while others who have even been diagnosed with the specific disease, often lack any presence of the virus.

If you think about it, what are the differences between strep throat, pharyngitis, Influenza, mononucleosis or Acute HIV syndrome? Or between Measles and Hand, Foot and Mouth disease? Even Polio is no different than any other disease accept for the paralysis and nervous system damage that was directly correlated to known poisons.

## The Theory in Practice

Vaccines are considered by the medical establishment to be the epitome of a modern-day miracle. They have been touted as the greatest discovery that man has achieved for Immune Health and the eradication of disease. That's what was declared about Jenner's Cowpox Vaccine. It is what is still declared by the CDC, WHO, HHS and in every medical school and hospital policy. For over 200 years, this theory of being able to train the body, by means of toxoids, attenuated and other viruses and bacteria, to grow (or build) antibodies against specific pathogens to protect against future outbreaks of disease, persists.

As we touched on at the beginning of this chapter, the ability of the body to create anti-bodies (white blood cells/ memory T cells, B cells etc.) is pretty much the entire "science" around which vaccines are built. If vaccines can help your body create a memory about disease, without actually giving the body the disease, that would, indeed, be a breakthrough, at least worth considering. Quite honestly, it's a beautiful sounding idea, one that made sense to me when I first read about it in my science and medical textbook. The problem is: it doesn't work the way they claim and there is nothing beautiful about vaccination.

The body does have the ability to create "immunity", which is really memory, against (or about) foreign entities that it has encountered before. If it didn't then I would never have had an issue with carrying a baby with a blood type (that carries a foreign protein) opposite mine. This "memory" is established in our blood, which is where the information and life of our whole system resides. Blood is a living substance that is actively oxygenating, energizing, cleansing, protecting and healing the body. Antibodies that are harvested from a host (usually mouse) are simply particles of that immune system. B cells (as best as we can identify them) taken from a host do not contain the same functional properties as they do while circulating in the blood or maturing in the spleen. Think about it as you would protein function.

Proteins in the body are made up of amino acids and are responsible for every repair and function of the body. They communicate with each other and every body part by hormone synthesis and actively create, heal and coordinate all aspects of bodily processes. "Protein" such as found in meat (the dead muscle and tissue mass of an animal) has (or had) all this material in it, but they are not actively building or healing the body, until the body takes the material provided and creates new proteins.

The B antibodies that are injected into you are attempted to be kept alive (such as in monoclonal antibody injections, which we will describe in greater detail later) by transforming (fusing) these cells into new cells that can be replicated (cloned).

There are many articles and studies that show that people who have the presence of very specific antibodies in their blood still get the diseases that they have been vaccinated for, in fact, it seems to increase the likelihood!

We will dive more into the theories and proofs of why in the next few chapters.

## The Disease Process

The body encounters non-self-entities every day. Most of these don't seem to cause a problem unless there is some caustic substance (or threatening element) involved. Proteins that contain pieces or parts of foreign materials (particularly of other living people or animals, insects etc.) can certainly be recognized by the body as elements to identify and dispose of. This would be the category that vaccines are attempting to replicate.

Bacteria that do not belong and are proliferating (i.e. spreading and multiplying) actively, is the definition of an infection. Signs of this would include:

Discoloration or redness

Swelling/Inflammation/Pain

Bad odor

Open sore or wound that is oozing

Yellow or brown drainage

Abscess or seeping Etc.

This process can sometimes spread: especially to weak or exposed areas. We call that contagion (or being contagious). It should be well understood by anyone who understands health or disease processes that the way to deal with any infection would be to cleanse the area. Isolate what cannot be cleansed and wait until the process goes away or is receding (healing).

In vaccination, they do the exact opposite.

Much of what people call sickness is a detox process.

Coughing

Sneezing

Breaking out in rashes

Swollen Lymph glands

Vomiting

Diarrhea

Fever or headache (can be due to other things)

Also included would be "allergens" or sensitivities that an individual would react to (which could be fine for someone else)

All of these are a result of the body being exposed to toxins or harmful substances that it is trying to get rid of. These "toxins" could be a great many things:

Lead, arsenic, bleach, acids, plastics and any number of poisons

Drugs, pesticides, herbicides, etc.

Non-food particles & Non-self entities

Foreign matter, diseased matter...

Bacteria and any micro-organisms that are not friendly to the body.

Another category is:

Informational coding and sound/radio waves/vibrations or frequencies...

EMFs, lasers, powerlines, and a great number of frequency-emitting machines.

A Third category would be a category we are newly learning about, and I will post an article on, near the end, in the Appendix section, which could be:

Exosomes, pheromones, energetic signatures and similar substances that would classify as: spreading harmful information that is replicating and being passed on to others through "vaccine shedding." This is a category we have not had to worry about before we introduced mRNA technology into people via the COVID vaccinations.

This third category may be the most important and imminent to the "illness" we are currently being bombarded with, and I encourage you to read the article posted at the end of this book to learn more about it. For now, let's continue with the science that has already been proven and the "science" (so called) that already should've been disproven.

# Vaccination ≠ Immunization

Provoking the body to produce an "anti-gen" or antibodies to a particular substance that is (supposedly) causing disease, has been shown to be a failing science. The idea that we can isolate specific germs or bacteria that cause disease and train the body to build up defense against them is faulty for several reasons:

#1 The number of microbes that exist is similar to, (or perhaps greater) than the number of animal and plant life that exist on earth. While most microbes have been shown to be beneficial in a healthy body, there are many that could prove harmful if our body is predisposed to infection, suffering from trauma or a weakened immune system etc. Microbes that are already proliferating an infectious or breakdown process is something we wouldn't want in or near us: like having feces or waste products in our food or dwelling etc.

The number and types of bacteria that could be associated with any disease process is likely too diverse to be able to identify consistently, and furthermore, bacteria that have been identified and shown to be present in those exhibiting a particular set of symptoms (such as in smallpox, diphtheria, pertussis etc.) have also been shown to be present in perfectly healthy individuals showing none of these symptoms. Keep in mind that the names created for these bacteria and their corresponding diseases were invented before we even had the technology (or understanding) to accurately find and label exact microbes. As Charles Creighton pointed out, we were barely able to differentiate but a few shapes: like rod-shaped, circular, or filamentous. There never was an exact "varicella bacteria" or Diphtheriae, or Pertussis germ etc. These were names given to the set of symptoms being noted in someone who was sick. The rest was all a theory, or illusion really, that somewhere in the diseased matter used to inoculate another person, was a particular entity (virus) causing the disease; and that that little entity was going to protect the person from future disease by merely exposing the immune system to it. In practice, though, this never worked, and only added to the toxic load of the body.

#2 Exposing someone, purposefully, to bad microbes or foreign matter, does not build the immune system, it only hurts it. While it is true that the body has the ability to train itself (and create an army of white blood cells etc.) to take out foreign invaders that it has seen before, there is (literally) no advantage to exposing it early or often and much damage can be done (often permanent) with the methods used for exposure. I.E. creating an open wound prone to infection, injecting of toxins into the bloodstream, or at the very least, breaching the skin and mucosal membranes. All this increases the vulnerability of the body.

Creating Trauma Doesn't Reduce Trauma!

You could liken the event of encountering a foreign substance, perhaps to a bad experience, like trauma, or bad situations or enemies that we want to try and avoid in the future, to protect ourselves. Suppose we even COULD find the exact culprit and create a replica (as with an "attenuated virus"), having a picture of a "bad person" or harmful event thrown at us, probably doesn't prove to be a very effective method of ensuring that our next encounter is bound to end with a successful combat. Similarly, when we try to train the body against disease, through exposure to a piece of bacteria or virus, it doesn't keep someone from getting sick. It also doesn't produce the dramatic effect we're after (immune response). So, they must make sure they truly anger the immune system until it finally responds. This would probably be akin to doing things to "rile somebody up" or truly traumatizing a child, to try to teach him or her that there are bad people in the world. The sad result is almost always (if not always) a traumatized child whose psyche is now less able to handle the "bad guys" of the world, and often develops other, or worse issues. Who would do that?! But this is actually very similar to what we are trying to do to the body, and sometimes, the body doesn't survive the trauma. As we've already talked about in the chapter on *Vaccines and Their Ingredients*, the elements we have used to "make the body angrier" or "put it on alert" (i.e. adjuvants...) has caused a vast amount of "trauma" to the human body that NEVER would've EXISTED otherwise. Also, as is mentioned in the study on measles in chapter 4 under MMR and later (in Ch.9), there are instances where the antigen specific antibody is found to be in the blood of a person and they STILL can get the disease, yet this would make perfect sense if one understood that disease is the body eliminating toxins and foreign matter from within.

Lastly, if the truth about disease is that it is a proliferation of misplaced or confused microbes (finding themselves in an acidic or injured environment), then the problem was never any particular microbes to begin with, but the sort of environment they could be found in. The remedy in this case would be to improve the environment, with cleanliness and better nutrition etc.

We have taken an idea, or theory about how we think the body equips itself against invaders, as though it is a mere machine that we can manipulate to function according to our own dictates. I believe we err, because we lack understanding about how the body truly functions. For one, the body is able to distinguish between itself and every other entity, because the information for its being and existence lies within every cell and extends to every aspect of its being, NOT because it has been trained with foreign objects. Support the body so that it can continue to effectively do its job. Disease is, after all, the state of a system that has either been poisoned or neglected. Or a process of detoxing what is foreign or unwanted. Fighting disease with disease, is like trying to clean off dirt with dirt. They don't "cancel each other out," it just makes the body dirtier.

The "science" used from the beginning of vaccine theory, was extremely un-scientific. Never was it proven to do the only two things it should've done if there was ever any real value in vaccination: namely, **make the immune system stronger, or protect the body against future disease**.

In Jenner's days, "success" was gaged by exposing a part of the body to diseased material, and not having it react a certain way (not producing the "general pustule"). In later days, "success" meant "producing an immune response" (getting the body to react). At its best, it was producing antibodies against particular foreign entities. Yet, as we have seen and will see later, in the posts and studies on measles, that even having antigen-specific anti-bodies (or particles) in their blood did not keep people from developing measles or any other diseases! Dr. Creigton rightly compared the belief of the idea of vaccination to a religious fervor. One that had no basis in any observable, repeatable or scientific principle. Never did "success" mean: less people dying from disease or getting sick. That was the CLAIM never the reality. It is STILL NOT the reality.

The THEORIES: like The Germ Theory of Disease (see Ch. 7) on which hung the perpetuation of the practice of Vaccination, began with a lie and were perpetuated by creating more false theories about how disease worked. To explain further, let's look at what happened before the theory of Vaccination, to another theory, which enabled the premise vaccination is built on.

# CHAPTER 7

## THE THEORY BEFORE THE THEORY

The results of a rivalry between two French scientists, Antoine Bechamp and Lois Pasteur, would forever alter the history of food and medicine, as well as the ideas of how people have envisioned the disease process. A book called, *Bechamp or Pasteur? A Lost Chapter in the History of Biology* originally written in 1923 by Ethel Hume, and *Pasteur: Plagiarist, Imposter The Germ Theory Exploded* published in 1942, by R.B. Pearson, should have dispelled both the popularity and the distorted ideas of Louis Pasteur.

What, you may ask, does this have to do with vaccines? It has to do with framing our perspective of disease to one where we can accept and fully embrace the lies of vaccination. The ideas that the more popular, but not more ingenious Pasteur, first stole from Antoine Bechamp, then twisted to support his own theories, (and, in some cases later resorted to admitting the truth of,) became the more widely accepted theories that persist today. In the words of the author, you will find in its pages, "convincing evidence that Pasteur discovered nothing, and that he deliberately appropriated, falsified and perverted another man's work.(Pearson p. 11)" More devastatingly, he proclaimed and published ideas that became foundations for hurtful medical practices, which we will discuss in this chapter.

For example, when the first well-known discovery of microbes came into the public realization, it was widely believed that these microbes, also termed “germs” by Pasteur, were the evils of the world to be blamed for every ill of man. We now know that microbial life is certainly not evil (at the very least they cannot all be), for they are in large part responsible both for our very existence and ability to thrive, including digesting and utilizing our food. When looking back in time, one can see that, from the very beginning, Bechamp had the right ideas about how these “little bodies (or microzymas)” as he called them, worked.

Bechamp conducted many series of experiments with fermentation, in which he proved that these little, unseen microbes, were always present, and an active part of the change of a substance into another by means of ingesting the sugars and other materials and leaving behind new by-products. You could think of it like what trees do for our oxygen supply.

We know that the leafy greens of plant life take in what we discard, namely CO2, and convert it into Oxygen, that we utilize to energize and renew our bodies. Similarly, Microbes take organic, discarded matter, whether plant or animal, and convert it into substances that can be reused as a part of new, living systems. This process happens when a plant breaks down and is disassembled by tiny microorganisms into more soil, which can be utilized as a medium for new plant growth. Microbes are part of every conversion process of our food, from milk becoming yogurt and cheese and yeasts and starter causing bread to rise. They are also responsible for every conversion of every life process, from renewing the soil to decomposing dead flesh.

The best way to describe these "little bodies" is to compare them to seeds and plants. Indeed, even the very tiniest single cell of a microbe can take nutrients (favorable to its particular needs) and water and become active and able to transform the materials around it. Large aggregates or colonies are established and proliferate much better. A well-nourished and well-established colony, like that of a well-formed SCOBY (symbiotic culture of bacteria and yeasts), has a greater ability to "culture" the liquid it's placed in, such as tea and sugar, and transform it into Kombucha, or other fizzy, cultured beverages. While we may not understand exactly how, we have witnessed the acts of these tiny microbes in just about every area of our life.

Rather like Dr. Charles Creighton, the accomplishments achieved by the end of Antoine Bechamp's life is rather astounding, and titles he earned include:

Doctor of pharmacy. Doctor of science. Doctor of Medicine. Professor of Medical Chemistry and Pharmacy at the Faculty of Medicine in Montpelier. Fellow and Professor of Physics and Toxicology at Higher School of Pharmacy at Strasbourg and Professor of Chemistry at the same town. Corresponding member of the Imperial Academy of Medicine of France and of the Society of Pharmacy of Paris. Member of the

Agricultural Society of Hirault and of the Linnaean Society of the department of Maine at Loire. Gold medalist of the industrial Society of Mulhouse (for the discovery of a cheap process for the manufacture of aniline and of many colors derived from this substance.) Silver medalist of the Committee of Historic Works and Learned Societies (for works upon the production of wine). Professor of Biological Chemistry and Dean of the Faculty of Medicine of Lille.
Honorary and titles include: Officer of Public Instruction, Chevalier of the Legion of Honor and Commander of the Rose of Brazil. (Ethel Hume p. 108-109)

A wealth of titles, yet, this biographer points out, in his own words, that "Antoine Bechamp was utterly indifferent to personal ambition. Never of a pushing temperament, he made no effort to seek out influential acquaintances and advertise his successes to them. Self-oblivious, he was entirely concentrated upon nature and its mysteries, never resting till something of these should be revealed ( Hume p. 111)."

Antoine Bechamp, indeed, shared that proficiency and love of science and nature itself that leads one to true discoveries of its mysteries. Pearson also said of him, "Bechamp's deep insight had taught him the connection between science and religion... and even his book: Les Microzymas, culminates in the acclamation of God as the Supreme source (p. 116)."

If you look into the little known and unadvertised stories of some of the greatest minds of the past, you would find a repeated, sad proliferation of men who could have made great contributions to the world, yet were squelched by want of recognition, control and power, and greed that chooses to silence the lives of brilliant scientists for the sake of gain. Time would prevent me from talking about the lives of brilliant men, like Royal Raymond Rife, whose intricate microscope and flawless technique, enabled him to make discoveries and declarations about the microscopic world (so far beyond that of Leeuwenhoek), that not only baffled and astounded the world of microbiology, but would've brought wondrous breakthroughs in science and medicine, had he not been silenced.

Such actions, laden with selfish ambition, from those who prefer thievery and power have left us with a history capable of exploiting and manipulating the masses for capital gain. Perhaps this is a history many would rather not be aware of, yet, if truth is not brought to light, freedom and justice cannot exist.

Now, we'll reflect on the works of Pasteur. For truly, Pasteur played his part in this arena of vaccines, as we'll soon see.

## The Creation of the Germ Theory of Disease

Three men: Geronimo Fracastorio (an Italian Poet and physician in 1483-1553) and M.A. Plenciz along with Antonius van Leenwenhoek, (discovery made in 1683), were the sources for Pasteur's theories. Fracastorio's *seminaria contagionum* were the culprits that he believed caused disease, either through immediate contact or through the air. These tiny microbes, he believed were capable of reproduction in the appropriate medium and "became pathogenic through the action of animal heat (R.B. Pearson p. 11)."

Leenwenhoek, a Dutch naturalist and lens maker, discovered the presence of, what he called, *animalcula,* which he described as rod-shaped and spiral-like and were later named, bacillus *buccalis maximus* and *spirillum sputigenum*. Later, in 1762, a Viennese physician named M.A. Planciz, published his *Germ Theory of Infectious Disease*. Plenciz asserted that there was a special organism responsible for each disease, that they were capable of reproducing outside the body, and that they could be passed on, or carried from person to person through the air. This theory was the bedrock for Pasteur's assertations, although he claimed to have "thought of it" and published the idea as his own (p. 12).

I find it astounding and refreshing that the famous and industrious Florence Nightingale published an attack on this theory, in 1860, over 17 years before Pasteur's claims. I want to record her ideas on this "germ theory" in her own words, because I believe her wisdom on the matter is quite valuable.

"Diseases are not individual classes, like cats and dogs, but connections growing out of one another.

Is it not living in a continual mistake to look upon diseases as we do now, as separate entities, which must exist, like cats and dogs, instead of looking upon them as conditions, like a dirty and a clean condition, and just as much under our control; or rather as the reactions of kindly nature, against the conditions in which we have placed ourselves?

I was brought up to believe that smallpox, for instance, was a thing in which there was once a first specimen in the world, which went on propagating itself in a perpetual chain of dissent, just as there was a first dog (or a first pair of dogs) and that smallpox would not begin itself, any more than a new dog would begin without there having been a parent dog. Since then, I have seen with my own eyes and smelled with my own nose smallpox growing up in first specimens, either in closed rooms or in overcrowded wards where it could not by any possibility have been caught but must have begun. I have seen diseases begin, grow up, and turn into one another. Now dogs do not turn into cats. I've seen for instance with a little overcrowding, continued fever grow up; and with a little more, typhoid fever and with a little more, typhus and all in the same ward or hut. Would it not be far better, truer and more practical if we looked upon disease in this light (for diseases, as all experience shows, are adjectives not noun substantives):

- True Nursing ignores infection, except to prevent it. Cleanliness and fresh air from open windows, with unremitting attention to the patient, are the only defense a true nurse either asks or needs.

- Wise and humane management of the patient is the best safeguard against infection. The greater part of nursing consists of preserving cleanliness.

- The specific disease doctrine is the grand refuge of the weak, uncultured, unstable minds such as now rule in the medical profession. *There are no specific diseases; there are specific disease conditions." (p.12-13)*

If ever there was someone who knew exactly what she was talking about and had firsthand experience in multitudes of disease conditions (and lived to tell of it) it was Florence Nightingale.

I truly hope to show, throughout this book, that the voice of reason has continued to go out into the world, but it has been largely silenced by incapable, degenerate, small minds who care more to protect their own ego, than to use one's gifts to serve humanity or proclaim truth.

Based on this belief: that every disease has a specific entity responsible for it, and that infecting a human system with a piece, part or replica of this entity, will guarantee, for life, protection from that particular disease, stems the practice of vaccination.

Pasteur, himself, participated in the vaccine hoax, by his contribution of the Anthrax serum and treatment protocol for rabies. When Pasteur heard a Frenchman named Delafond proclaim, in 1838, that there were little rod-shaped objects found in the blood of animals that had splenic fever or charon (which we now call Anthrax), he declared, "Anthrax is, therefore, the disease of the bacteridium, as trichinosis is the disease of the trichina, as itch is the disease of its special acarus (p.61)."

So quick was he at making such a judgment call. Here, we see the circular theorizing of calling specific diseases (or disease processes) after the name, they declared, of specific bacteria.

It's been said, that one of the characteristics of bacteria (or microbes) is that they have the ability to change (or morph) into different forms, based on the sort of environment they are found in. I think it's more likely that certain kinds of microorganisms just don't "take hold" or don't grow, until the environment becomes more favorable (mirroring what we see in the natural world). Either way, the observable phenomenon is that "bad microbes," if there is such a thing, simply do not cause a problem to a healthy, living system. Perhaps much like maggots "spontaneously erupting" on the underbelly of a decaying animal, these microorganisms aggregate in places they feel called, or drawn, to act on. Of course, I use the idea of maggots intentionally, while pointing out that this is a phenomenon we all know to be impossible. But the idea of Spontaneous Generation was invented by Pasteur, though it was later disproved.

If I could make a statement I believe to be true, "as it is in the observable creation, so is the unobservable." In other words:

"the unseen reflects the seen" so that what we cannot see, mirrors the same created order that one can behold and measure (like in a garden). These little (seemingly indestructible) beings can remain dormant both in harsh conditions and for apparently unlimited lengths of time. Then, these dormant seed pockets come to life when called upon, or when the conditions they find themselves in signal this transformative growth process. There could, after all, be literally millions of various "seed pockets" on any given surface at almost any given time, and these would also be able to transport through the air.

One thing we do know, is that when a large aggregate, or colony of organisms are found on a particular surface: such as in the face of death, these microorganisms can pass on their "active death process" to another organism, even another person. This is why contact with one person who has this process active somewhere on their body, can spread this "Death Process" to someone else, particularly if that person is wounded, vulnerable or compromised. This is why doctors who were handling dead bodies and then assisting with births, were unwittingly causing the deaths of women because of the contamination. When the doctors simply washed their hands first, the rates of death of these women from "childbirth" dropped dramatically. We are all quite familiar with this story, yet the profundity escaped doctors of that era because, with all their supposed knowledge and skill, they misunderstood this very basic concept of cleanliness. In the case of a dead body, the amount of, not just dormant, but active destructive (or decaying) microbes is profound (or abundant) and these microbes can "infect" another person, especially if there is a cut or wound or other compromise or weakness to the individual exposed.

Other disease processes work similarly. This is the case with disease processes that are "contagious." Contagion is a real thing, but it does not work the way many people picture the process in their mind. There is no "mysterious, unseen germ (or virus)" that causes the disease, rather, there is a spreading of the disease process in systems that are already compromised. This process can occur inside the body of a person (with absolutely no outside contact) when the PH drops low enough, or the energy flow becomes too dis-resonant, or a part of the body gets an infection that continues to grow etc. Overall, the reasons that someone "gets sick" or suffers from a disease, are complicated and highly variable, and most often there are compounding levels (or degrees) of compromise that prime the body for sickness or infection. Such factors could include bad diet, stress, trauma, poisoning, lack of oxygen, stagnation, chronic internal dissidence, weakness in a part of the body, genetic pre-dispositions, exhaustion and many other things.

## The Anthrax Vaccine

Because Pasteur, as many believed in that era, purported that particular microbes cause disease, he further proposed the idea that both toxins and "antitoxins" could be the key to irradicating all diseases. Pasteur attempted to create a vaccine with "tamed anthrax bacteria" or "less virulent" ones. He believed that "aerobic germs" were the Bacillus (or bacteria itself) and that "anaerobic germs" were the cause of "putrefaction", not a condition brought on by filth or compromise. Somehow, all this led him to believe that if he combined the two: aerobic and anaerobic germs, that this would neutralize the effects (or virulence) of the bacillus, and that when injected with this substance, the animal would be protected (p.61). Interestingly, this is the same phrase we use to describe our (neutralizing) antibodies today! Dr. Colin (physician) challenged Pasteur's statement saying that Anthrax was sometimes found in its virulent stage, and yet unaccompanied by the "bacteridia" (just like now). Also, he made a statement that the anthrax bacteria did not develop in sheep that were "healthy." There was also another inconsistency of the declaration that some of their sources of anthrax would produce continual amounts of the rod-shaped bacteria, consistently delivering all the same symptoms. Yet, the only bacteria produced from the batch was a little circular one that didn't even cause sickness (p.62). Apparently, these bacteria that produce when and where they're "supposed to" (or called upon in the natural world) are not so easy to control, manipulate or proliferate at will. Or perhaps the problem remains that it is not the little bacteria that "cause" the disease in the first place.

However, sadly, we HAVE succeeded, now, in proliferating both antigens (diseased/ foreign particles) and antibodies (or the little pieces we harvest from a mouse's spleen).

There were many injuries and deaths because of the vaccinations. Injecting substances into animals was causing numerous other diseases and problems. An outbreak of lethal hoof and mouth disease spread in an area that was previously vaccinated. This disease, while troublesome, rarely killed the animal it infected. In the vaccination cases, this disease became quite serious. By 1902 and 1908, the outbreaks were most severe. Many herds of animals, both infected and exposed, had to be slaughtered and buried to effectively eradicate the disease. At an institute in Russia, 3,696 sheep of the total 4,564 that were vaccinated with Anthrax "preventative" promptly died (p.66). This is over 80%. While Pasteur was compelled to compensate many owners in France for the loss of their animals, he still continued his work.

The secretary of Agriculture was quoted as stating that, "Up to the present time the germ (of hoof and mouth disease) has not been identified, although the scientists of Europe have studied the disease exhaustively for years."(p, 69) Hmmm, I wonder how that's possible??

In the 1914-1915 epidemic, 168,158 animals were killed worth around $5,676,000 to suppress the disease. As unbelievably profound as this was, Pasteur's treatment plan for rabies is perhaps even more disturbing.

## A Real History of Rabies

I remember, vividly a movie that portrayed a man, who, supposedly contracted rabies after being attacked by a dog, in a most disturbing and eerie way. The reality, I believe, is so less dramatic. In fact, there are studies that beg to differ with purported beliefs, and claims that rabies is contractual from a rabid dog, even if that dog bites you. The madness of a dog who behaved so erratically seemed to be more related to a disease in their bowels that erupts, causing them to behave unseemly, lash out, foam at the mouth etc. (Pearson p.72) The more recent rusty nail phobia, is also likely overexaggerated, and I do find it rather worth noting that I've never known, or even heard of anyone, ever, contracting rabies from stepping on... anything... ever.

Regardless, though, as one ought to, by now, expect, Pasteur's "treatment" caused profound problems. The inoculations, which were designed to "prevent rabies" actually caused a condition referred to as Hydrophobia (Rabies). Taken from the word, which literally means a fear of water, this "late stage symptom of rabies" as they called it, causes convulsions and an inability to drink water due to the thrashing, (but also difficulty to swallow) caused by CNS damage. There never was a case of either "hydrophobia" or "rabies" from a dog bite until it was proposed as the cause by over 3,000 people who died after they were bit by (supposedly infected) dogs and consequently vaccinated with Pasteur's serum.(p.73) During the same time, "2,668 persons bitten by dogs were treated without using Pasteur's treatment" at a hospital in London, none of which developed "Hydrophobia." This info doesn't include the thousands of dogs which were killed due to the scares.

So, it seems, "rabies" is a scam, and a deflection of blame for a disease directly caused by the "treatment." After researching the topic more thoroughly, the nonsense (more like non-existence) of the mysterious rabies infections are more unsubstantiated than I ever imagined. While it is true that if you injure yourself (by whatever means or object) and an infection persists (due to neglect or ineffective treatments) to the point where nervous system, brain, organ, or other serious damage can occur, one could experience epilepsy, convulsions, and a wide variety of serious issues, even leading to death. This rarely occurs, though, but happens far more often as a result of vaccine poisoning.

Let's move on to the place where our first histories of the infamous smallpox vaccination and Pasteur meet. Whether or not one could consider Pasteur and Jenner "friends," they certainly were embarked on similar ambitions in the world of medicine, as can be seen by the books by Charles Creighton and Ethel Hume, and thanks to the exploitation and popularization of the "Germ Theory of Disease," the practice and compulsion of vaccination continue to this day.

## More charts and Graphs

Here are more charts and statistics that prove how deaths from disease, and particularly smallpox, rise substantially due to vaccination (Pearson p.77).

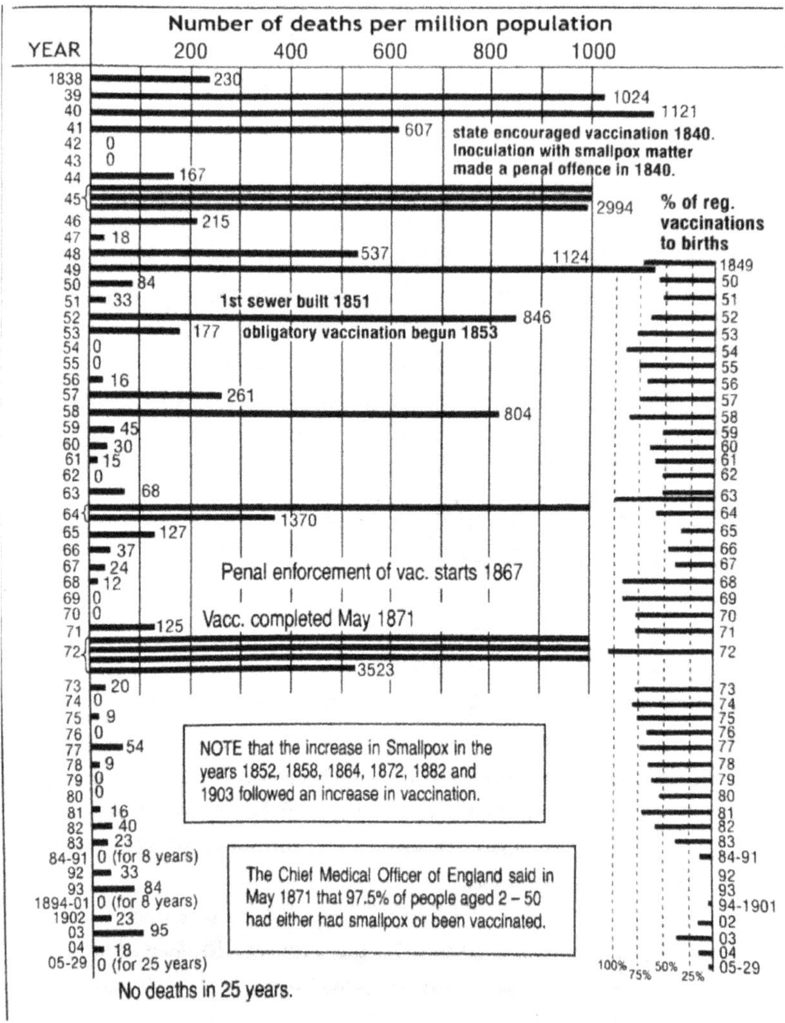


**Smallpox and Vaccination in Leicester, England**

Note how every increase in vaccination as indicated in the lines in the right-hand column was followed by an increase in the smallpox death rate.

The worst epidemic came in 1872, following the most extensive, four-year effort to have complete vaccination. The Medical officer announced that 97.5% of the population had either had smallpox or been vaccinated.

In contrast, during the years from 1905 to 1938, the public had so lost confidence in vaccination that less than 6% of newborns were vaccinated for about a 20-year period. It is very notable that during that time, for 33 years, there were no recorded deaths from smallpox.

As noted in the British Medical Journal on Jan. 14th, 1928, Dr. R. Garrow, Medical Officer of Health for Chesterfield, England asked "Why it is that the case mortality rate from smallpox in all persons over the age of 15 in England and Wales for the years 1923-1926 was five times as high in the vaccinated as in those who were unvaccinated!"(p. 76)

From my own observation of the previous graph, the era of the 1950s seems to me the least consistent (considering the harshness of the vaccine law mandate) but also follows a time where a huge uprising was made against the compulsory law (as we see from these recorded histories) and also followed a great improvement in plumbing. While we do see a huge surge in deaths right after the compulsory law was established, the numbers marvelously decrease. Perhaps the cries of insurrection were successful after all. At least for awhile.

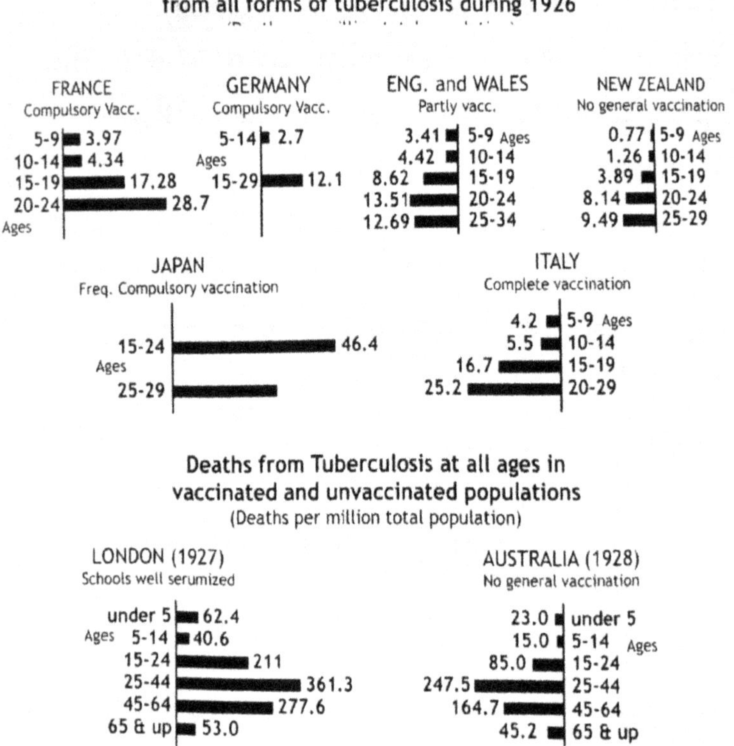


### Vaccines and Tuberculosis at School Ages

Note how much higher the death rate is in countries having compulsory vaccination, such as Japan and Italy, than in countries without compulsion, such as England, Wales and New Zealand. (p.80)

As we discussed earlier, Tuberculosis, is a secondary infection due to contaminating the system with vaccines, also known as biologicals, and was rampant among inoculated individuals.

Vaccines and Other Diseases

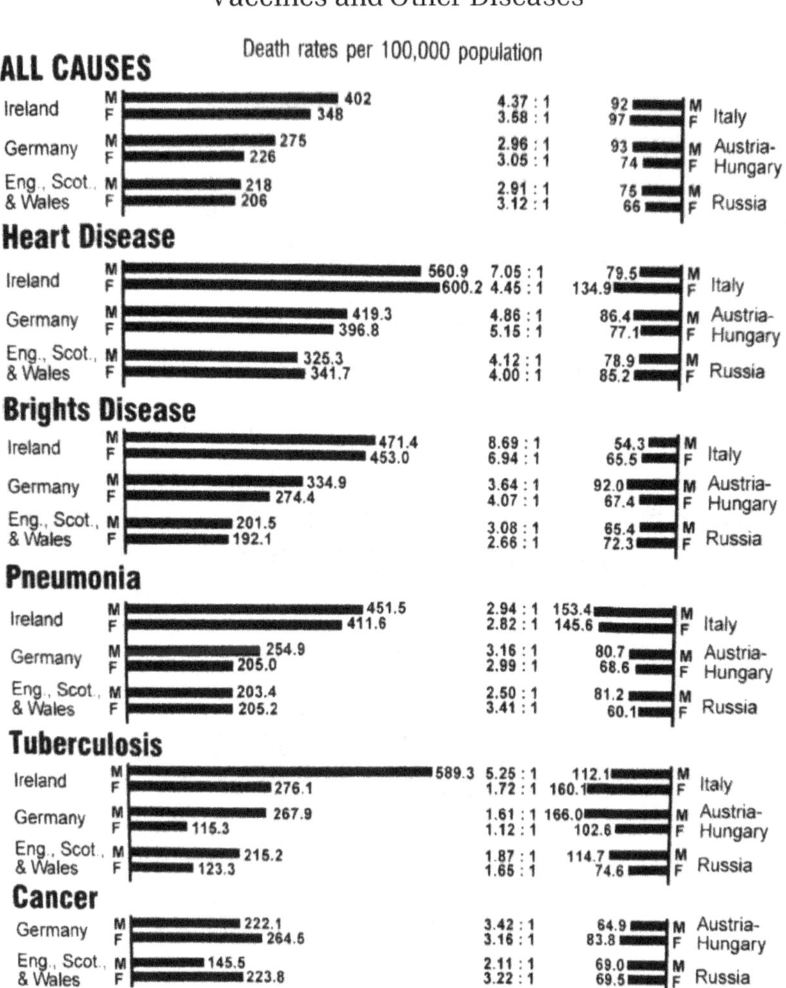


**Mortality from highly fatal diseases among various groups of immigrants in New York State in 1910**

Note that much higher death rates prevail among migrants from countries having compulsory vaccination (left side of diagram) than among immigrants from countries without compulsion (right side). (p.81)

As noted before, the development of other diseases is certainly increased when vaccination is practiced.

While I'm not going to mention every chart or statistic in this book, I feel compelled to add at least one more. Similar figures, as those in previous diagrams, show increases in cases of scarlet fever, Diphtheria and Croup in England and Wales, which cases drop substantially after 1871, with the exception of Diphtheria, which actually increases after 1893: a seven-year period in which Diphtheria anti-toxin was being heavily pushed. (p.84)

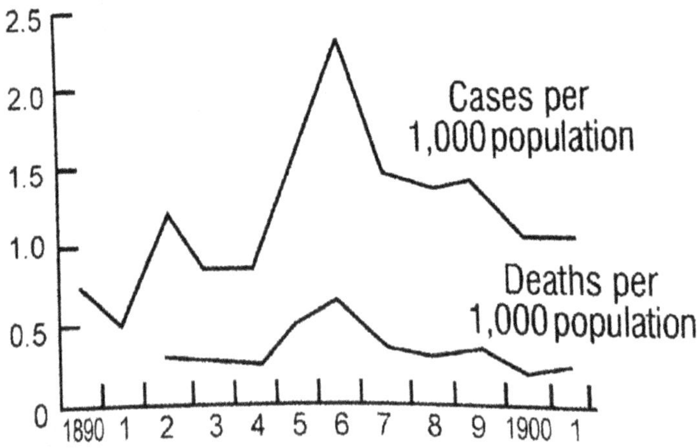


**Diphtheria in Birmingham, 1890 to 1901**

From the report of the Health Officer for Birmingham, 1901.

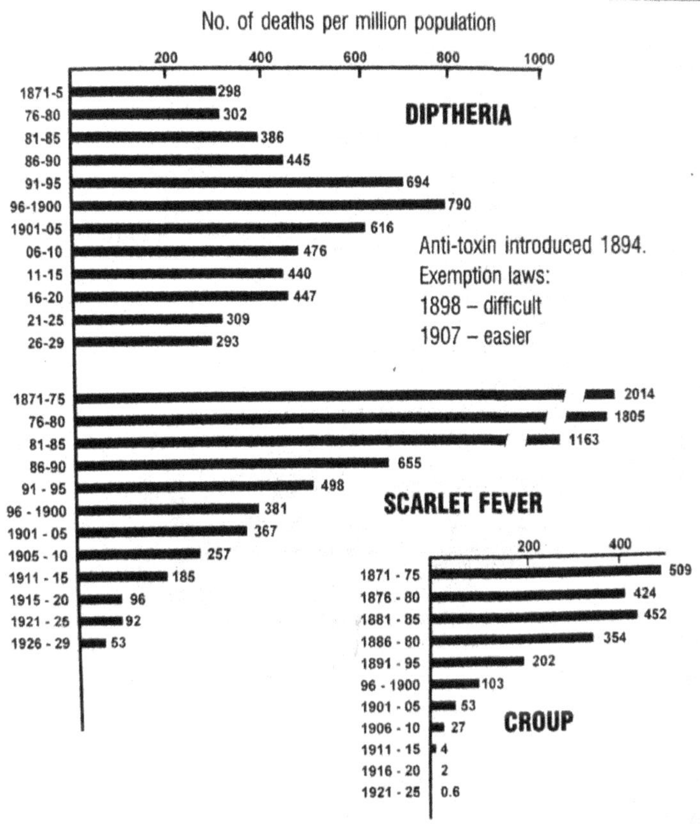


**Diphtheria, Scarlet Fever and Croup in England and Wales.**

"Note how the diphtheria death rate was held up well above the 1871 to 1880 rate ever since anti toxin was introduced in 1893, while the death rates from scarlet fever and croup have consistently gone down at a rapid rate without the use of any biological."

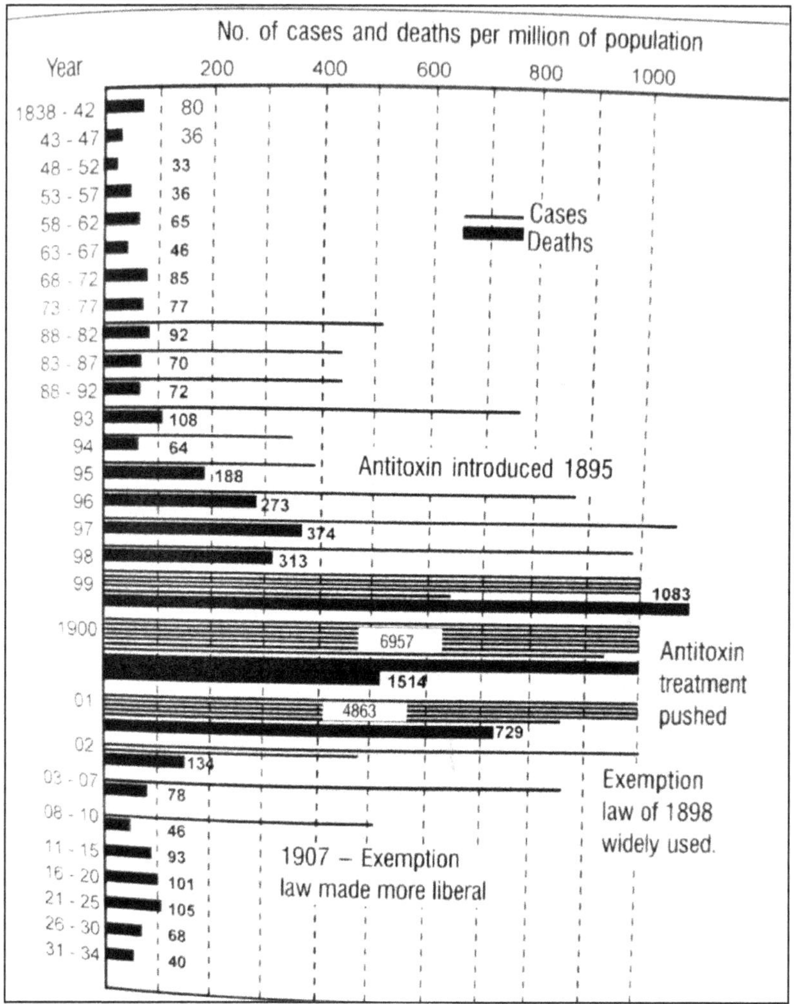


**Diphtheria in Leicester England -cases and deaths**

Note how sharply the death rate rose after antitoxin was introduced in 1895 from an average of 62 per year for the previous 57 years to a high of 1514 deaths in 1900. (p.87)

I find it most disturbing, that after studying diphtheria more closely for the purposes of writing this book, I'm amazed that they are still, not only offering diphtheria vaccine but also encourage antitoxin to those who seem to be experiencing symptoms. While the reasons given are to "prevent organ damage," it seems obvious that the reverse would be true. I can completely imagine a scenario where such an antitoxin could cause serious damage, even leading to death, and it would be excused, or blamed rather, on the "Disease itself" rather than the toxins being used in the supposed protection against it.

**In conclusion**: None of these histories, charts or graphs proved the prevention of disease or increase in health of any of the recipients. In fact, the exact opposite has been and still is proven repeatedly. Especially now that we have an ever-increasing amount of vaccines being recommended, it should be noted that disease and damage increase with every vaccine dose given.

I do wish we would learn from our mistakes in history and finally stop this medical evil and human injustice. Pearson quotes Dr. Leverson's strong and passionate statement on the matter that, "the forcing of these inoculations upon individuals by law is one of the worst tyrannies imaginable and should be resisted even to the death of the official who is enforcing it." (p.41)

If this were the protocol that had been carried out, the prevention of so much untold misery and death could have been prevented. The continued practice of inoculation/ vaccination is an utterly unnecessary and horrifically harmful "treatment" protocol. It is my heart desire that this evil could be eradicated from our entire medical system and future moving forward, but if not, then my desire is to at least educate as many as I can so that this evil does not forever impact or devastate the families of those reading this, or whose ears are blessed to receive the truth.

The thing to be feared is not the microorganisms that we cannot see, and the disease process itself is not a condition being unwittingly thrust upon helpless victims, no, the evil to revolt against is the defilement of the human body and the blood and the brain, and every internal, sacred part by forcing toxins and foreign material into it!

# CHAPTER 8

## WHAT IS A VIRUS?

While we have talked at length about the idea of bacteria, germs and other microorganisms, we have not really discussed the matter of viruses. Viruses are, after all, the entities supposedly responsible for so many disease processes. They are the reason we vaccinate, as well as the entities used to vaccinate with.

When the COVID-19 "epidemic" hit, I began researching viruses, realizing my own idea was probably far from an accurate one. While the area of microbiology was one of my favorite things to read about and study, I felt hit by the sudden realization (in 2019) that I had no idea what a virus really was. I'd always thought that they were microorganisms like bacteria, only smaller (or something like that) but with so much rage and blame being put on viruses, I felt the need to solidify the definition in my own mind. Partially because how the media was alluding to viruses wasn't making much sense.

I read books by virologists, particularly Plague, by Judy Mikovitz. That one I read in its entirety! And, while the story was riveting and exciting etc. I think I was at least ¾ of the way through, before I felt I had an actual, concrete definition of what a virus was, according to a virologist.

So, here is my take:

First of all, it may be helpful to define what a virus is Not. It is NOT a LIVING organism. It is Not a Germ. Not a human, or other living being's cell. It is not a living microbe or other kind of organism at all.

It is a fraction, or section of DNA or RNA material, wrapped in a "protein package." Or, as a scientist might say, "one nucleic acid strand (DNA or RNA genes) and one protein capsule."

What does that mean? If you're like me, you might say, "that does not give a full or clear picture of its significance", or answer the questions, "Where do they come from? What do they do? Why are they a problem?" Etc.

It is a fact that viruses show up pretty much everywhere people are sick (I would say, detoxing). In other words, if you are sneezing, coughing, breaking out, feeling ill, experiencing inflammation etc. you will find these snippets nearby. Now, the fact that they are literal "snippets" of DNA or RNA, often your own; one might wonder why that's a problem. Well part of what makes these little pieces of strands significant is they're jumbled, out of order, chaotic or just foreign code snippets that either don't come from the cell, are from our cells but get twisted or distorted somehow, or might, in some cases, be pieces of code just like our DNA but the cell doesn't need them, perhaps like extras. It's also significant to point out that EVERY LIVING THING that has a DNA code, offshoots viruses. That is pretty much the summary "scientific" definition of what a virus is.

However, since the word, VIRUS is a part of our language and used for many things that stand outside the "scientific recognition," we may need to expand our definition.

While viruses definitely operate in the world of information particles, one could think of a virus as: information that exists and can reinforce, alter or change the identity, substance or function of a cell or system. If accepted and used by that system then the cells of the body can replicate these "protein packages" (really information packages) enough to cause a serious problem. It could even change the very structure or essence of our being. Why the body, or our cells, would want to accept this alternate "code of reality" could be another substantial question to ponder.

In this regard, you could look at the definition of a virus as being **false information.** With this definition, one could say that ALL sickness stems from viruses.

In regarding DNA functions, while we might not fully understand all the nuances, we know they are informational: DNA literally holds the information for our entire existence. Every living being on planet earth has a genetic code that holds the information of its being and essence.

If this is the reality, then it makes sense that during certain seasons, when plants and other life forms are shedding their own "viruses" that when we breathe them in etc., we are more likely to exhibit some sort of detox reaction, as millions of these, non-us, particles are being shed and eliminated at an increased rate. In normal healthy humans, though, the informational particles in our natural world would be known to us and not pose any threat. The increase in the types of diseases and detoxing happening lately is certainly not natural.

When our body (or cell) is bombarded by any sort of toxin, or even an injury, or food particle (particularly where it doesn't belong) or any caustic substance (or any substance that causes us to react negatively), or radiation, even certain vibrations or sound waves, or even negative talk, curses or trauma etc. could cause a beak or disruption in the normal transcription of DNA in our cells. Now, not all genes are the same, and some are designed to be more fluid and easily influenced, such as epigenetics, while others are more firmly stable and need to be in order to preserve our existence.

The rate at which our being is continually decoding and reassembling these miles of information, flawlessly, happens at an astounding rate. The precision with which this happens is nothing short of miraculous. Tiny fragments that become extra or distorted are rarer than you might think, but likely happen all the time and our body just disposes of these fragments or re-assembles the amino acids and proteins without a problem.

Now, it used to be that vaccination dealt, primarily, with a diseased matter that they infected people with. As we stated before, you can't fight disease, with disease, or filth with filth, but now, we are fighting another "unseen" battle, when we are dealing with viruses. Our ideas of bacteria have changed quite a bit from the old days of blaming them as mysterious predators for the ills we experience, and we have seen the decrease in many of the earlier diseases simply by cleanliness and better living conditions. Now, we have a "new unseen evil": viruses. Now we vaccinate against "viral diseases." Something with a far broader implication, and that is even more mysterious. You could literally create an idea of a disease in people's minds or look at any kind of health problem or set of symptoms, blame it on a "virus" and then create a vaccine (or pharmaceutical cure) to combat it. What if there isn't any such thing?? Or at least, not the way it's being painted to the public. While viral fragments on their own don't pose any lethal threat to a person, the information we are being fed and injected with come along with a host of problematic and lethal substances.

Our cells, like us, are social creatures. (This is just one way of looking at it.) Drop a microbe or a virus in a healthy person and it doesn't stand a chance. Incorporate a significant amount of microbes that are actively growing disease and now you have a battle on your hands. A battle that the body may or may not be successful at fighting off. Likely, this is exactly the sort of battle we are seeing emerge with viruses. Multiply the false/ harmful informational patterns enough and we won't stand a chance.

Fill the world with every kind of herb, tree and animal that carries its own DNA code and place a person into it and they will thrive and learn to recognize the foreign entities (if you could even call them that) as friends to their existence. Disrupt the flow with distorted information, toxins, disruptors, and all kinds of invaders causing us harm and the body can only handle the bombardment to a certain extent.

I think we would find, at the very root of our present illnesses, the problem to be false information. The degree to which we are able to withstand this influx is the degree to which we know ourselves, properly and can distinguish between good and evil. In purely physical terms, you could say, it is the amount of false information we are able to withstand and eliminate with a good, working immune system. The reasons for accepting or allowing false information to "take root" and begin to shape or alter our design and function, could be simply (and quite broadly) the amount of false information being thrust upon us or the weakened state we may find ourselves in.

## A Problem Bigger than Measles

I found it very interesting (as we read about earlier) that in Corpus Christi, TX in 1983, where there were 400 students that had been vaccinated (98% vaccination rate) that 97% of these, shown to have antibodies (memory antibodies) still got measles! During the Jennerian era of vaccination, not breaking out in a "general pustule" was the way they gaged "success" (or protection), now we have the ability to test the blood and see that there are "memory antibodies" that have developed in a person's immune system. This means that the body has been shown to remember (or reacted to) these particles (particles from the vaccine) in the disease, yet these same people came down with all the symptoms of measles. If this is true, then how can anyone ever justify vaccinating against such a disease?? Or any disease? Is it not extremely profound to realize that injecting foreign matter into someone, that alerts the immune system, and leaves it scared enough to be on the alert for these foreign entities, does NOTHING to STOP the DISEASE PROCESS?! I think this means we need a new theory of disease.

Now, in the case of measles, it is certainly notable (and should be perfectly understandable) that the live virus (which is actually living bacteria in diseased tissue) vaccine **causes** the measles outbreak, like Gregory Poland, the vaccinologist at the Mayo Clinic, stated in his *Paradox of Measles*, saying that "you cannot eradicate a virus like measles with a live virus, due to shedding," along with the proof that measles did, indeed, develop in vaccinated individuals at a substantially higher rate than unvaccinated. Such was the case in the 2015 measles outbreak at Disney in California.

So, in the case of measles, we are injecting living, infectious matter (microbes) into someone, and that is likely to create an infection the body will (hopefully) try to detox.

In the case of pretty much every other vaccine (but this is also the case with MMR), the worst problem is not the diseased material as much as the other, more caustic and more dangerous ingredients (like adjuvants such as mercury and aluminum), which can cause brain damage, CNS damage, organ damage, and with the mRNA technology, now possible lasting and permanent damage (change) to the DNA itself. With an extended definition of "virus" you could consider every caustic agent, including the adjuvants as viruses, since they are certainly foreign substances that disrupt normal processes in the cell, but more accurately, the adjuvants are concrete substantives (elements) that break down our cell's defenses like a catapult, plunging through cell membranes and blood brain barriers to open the door for other viral agents (like mRNA) and disease to wreak havoc.

Adjuvants are placed in vaccines for the express PURPOSE of creating alarm or STIMULATING a RESPONSE in the immune system. As we stated before, our new definition for "success" in vaccination is: producing an immune response, as well as measuring the amount of "antigen-specific (neutralizing) antibodies" to judge whether a person was successfully "immune" or not. Yet, even with our most advanced methods for determining whether someone has built immunity (anti-bodies) to specific elements of disease or pathogens, none of these confirmations keeps the individual from further contamination, disease processes or damage when exposed to more toxins. Only, the way we vaccinate now typically goes beyond any visible or typical disease or detox process, as the damage being done is on a much deeper level.

The Mayo Clinic describes measles as a "red blotchy rash usually appearing on the face and behind the ears and then down towards the chest and back and can even spread to the feet." Other symptoms would be "fever, cough, runny nose, sore throat, possible spots inside the mouth and perhaps inflamed eyes or conjunctivitis." All these are detox reactions.

I feel compelled to tell a personal story, since it is so timely and in line with the writing of this book. I have, very recently, experienced several severe detox reactions, which began with swelling around my eyes (which only lasted a day) to a very distinct rash (lasting several days) the most debilitating of which was pain and swelling in my hands, feet and joints. The rash was so much like a measles rash, my mother-in-law was convinced it was measles (or rubeola) and that I had picked it up somewhere. Nothing in my experience lined up with this hypothesis since we had just come back from a camping trip with multitudes of other families: none of whom experienced the same symptoms. However, I had several reasons to believe that my body was trying to detox. After nearly four years of prolonged hospital stays, procedures and surgeries (and yes, pharmaceuticals, anesthesia and even blood transfusions), on the journey of having my last two babies. Now, being 10 mo. postpartum, in the heat of summer, more active etc. I do believe that my body was trying to eliminate some toxins that had stored in my tissues, and that taking teas and other herbs etc. to try and help the process may have put my body into a detox mode that was a bit more than I could handle all at once. One thing I have learned about toxins and trauma is that the body can only deal with so much at a time. For some, the process of dealing with past trauma, or toxin build up can take years of recovery. For myself, I had noticed that I broke out in skin rashes and was extra sensitive to things (even the sun) more so than I ever had been, particularly since my last C-sect. and stay in hospital. So, to me, even though the issues may have seemed troublesome and baffling, it was really no surprise, since I knew I had much going on, and felt thankful that my body was working appropriately to deal with things as it was designed to. Disease, after all, is a process of your body attempting to deal with a problem. It was never meant to last forever. In my case, everything subsided in less than two weeks, though its peak was quite concerning and painful.

If "measles" and other (specific and non-specific) diseases is simply a detox reaction by the body to eliminate toxins, then it doesn't make any sense to contaminate it to try and protect it. A theory that would hold truer to reality is that every foreign object, pathogen, poison or trauma should be avoided as much as is reasonably possible, and that fortifying the immune system with nutrients, God-given, living agents and helping the body to detox is the way to faster healing.

When my little boy was about a year old, he had a sore throat, runny nose, broke out in a skin rash and had a fever. While I wouldn't have called it that, I'm pretty sure you could have diagnosed him as having a light or some sort of case of measles. I have seven children and remember most of my children having a similar detox reaction around the same age. Typically, children don't have the same type of skin reactions as they grow older and their systems mature, but that doesn't mean it's impossible.

I want you to know, this isn't just something I came up with on the fly, or only something I read or something someone told to me. I have deeply considered and tested the ideas now proclaimed in the medical industry, and I'm telling you, they just don't add up. Not in real life situations.

Whether little children (who get breakouts typically when they are young) seem to get them more seldomly when older, is due to their systems being more fragile and transparent, and apt to react more visibly; or whether it is due to their systems being trained to better and more efficiently [when they're older] deal with bacteria that they have become accustomed to, I don't think matters. The reality demonstrates that children who are exposed to their natural environment at an early age develop stronger immunity and a body better able to cope with the world around it, than a body that is either too neglected or too damaged. Vaccines help only with the damage part. It is my overwhelmingly firm belief that the greatest help you can offer your child is to strengthen their immunity and protect them from disease by feeding them a healthy diet, loving them, playing with them, laughing with them, taking them outside, into nature, to the water etc. and protecting them from harm. If you want to help train their immune system to develop antibodies to foreign substances, then support their immune system's ability to do this by building it up not tearing it down. It would be far better, at least less deadly, to let them roll around and eat dirt (non-GMO), than to inject them with toxins or biologicals of any kind!

**The Viral Theory Persists**

Now they are talking about the supposed "devastation that would result from our removing all vaccines from medical practice." I listened to Dell Bigtree give a sensible sounding speech about how we need to be methodical about how we deal with the area of vaccines. The hype about measles was the catalyst. The idea is that if we just remove them altogether, we will have a disaster on our hands of "unprotected littles who have never been exposed to measles before." I am appalled that he used the age group that would experience the most devastation and repercussions from vaccine damage. As though there is anything to be gained by unnecessarily exposing our babies to injected, harmful substances, rather than let them be exposed to their environment naturally: the way God intended. In a way that will allow them to keep their immune systems and health intact. This presupposition comes from a misunderstanding of the way disease works.

There is no virus causing the disease of measles! (though the word "virus" is up for an enormous amount of interpretation) **Measles** is a **name** for a **detox reaction** to substances that one is exposed to that produces a breakout, or rash in the skin (among other things). Not all detox reactions, not all symptoms are the same, but they are all a similar process. Not all toxins, biologicals, chemicals etc. cause the same effects in one person as they do another, and there are multiple reasons for this: one person may have a particular weakness that another doesn't, some people are genetically predisposed to react or be affected by certain substances, including certain types of foods; there can be multiple factors at play, including state of mind or stress level at the time of exposure, that all contribute to the impact on the body, as well as the body's ability to deal with it.

This is why not all people seem to be impacted the same from vaccinations. Some may not show any visible signs of problems or issues and there are some who may not have been vaccinated but given a placebo (I've read articles of this being the case with some of the COVID injections). Either way, the vaccines, themselves are certainly not all created equal. Some people may be affected or have damage that shows up later or impacts the body's ability to deal with stress, or contributes to allergies etc.

The truth is that no baby on earth (or human being on earth) will be negatively impacted by the absence of vaccines. On the other hand, the continued administration of them IS going to have lasting effects that will eclipse anything we've seen before. This is not something to be taken lightly or ignored.

## The Vaccine of the Future?

There is a new and growing agenda in the world of vaccines, and that is not just contamination, but alteration.

Contamination, as bad as that has been, is not nearly as devastating as alteration, because once your genes have been altered, the effects are not just long lasting, but ongoing, and can, and will, affect futures of generations. Just as the idea of putting known toxins into the body can never make it better but only make it worse; so, the idea that altering your genetic code (or information) will not only hamper your body's ability to function but distort your ability to be a fully functioning human.

I believe there will be a new and "different" kind of Vaccine that promises to be the most revolutionary gift of medicine we've seen yet. "Breakthroughs" in genetics will promise to be the answer for "fixing" a vast array of "debilitating diseases" using your own, personalized genetic biology information, and will promise to deliver "specialized treatments" also promised to be "safer and more revolutionary" than any before. Combining the power and efficiency of AI and technologies that supersede any we've seen before, along with the ability to detect and code for a great number of "genetic predispositions" that can then be specifically targeted, corrected and then redefined to intricately obliterate all malformations and genetic insufficiencies. This would be a technology that uses the dangerous technique of mRNA's ability to replicate a prescribed gene, literally transforming you into a "super human" or perhaps more accurately, sub or trans human. Redefining the very essence of what it means to be human.

Movies and stories of genetically altered "super-humans" are abundant but are a lie (and I do believe this will be the next lie that will allow the proliferation of a new and more devastating "vaccine" to continue). Altering someone's genes does not improve them; they always get worse. I know there are scientific studies and efforts in genetics to correct genetic malformation which, in theory, might succeed in improving someone's health and ability to function, and this would be the most delicate sort of operation of all, since it would be so easy to disrupt this complex code and produce an unknown array of ramifications.

However, in vaccines that use mRNA (or any other) technology to introduce or alter genetic code (to make it different than its original design) the results will only be negative, and negative to an astounding degree. One that we probably can't even comprehend at present.

## Monoclonal Antibodies

While much of what was just stated is still theoretical and futuristic (stated more as caution than present reality), what we

ARE seeing NOW, which could be the doorway to such possible developments, is in the field of Monoclonal Anti-bodies (mAbs). Most specifically: Hybridoma technology. An article on PubMed Central states, "This discovery is considered one of the most important turning points in the field of biotechnology."

## What are these Antibodies and how are they made?

In a basic summary: a host (like a mouse) is injected with high amounts of antigens (specific foreign entities) for a couple, or several weeks. Then the spleen of the animal is cut out and the B-cells harvested and isolated using technologies as centrifugation and ELISA. The cells are then joined with myeloma (cancer) cells or a part of them with the ability to replicate ad infinitum. These new cells are fused using substances like Polyethylene Glycol and are heterokaryon (have two nuclei) or can be fused electrically. Few cells survive this process, but the few that do are then replicated (or cloned).

Some of the problems with these hybridomas are that the cells being harvested do not live long (at most a few days) so they must be transfused into these other cells to perpetuate their lifespan and be cloned. At the very least, the downsides of this procedure is the infusion of unknown (and unavoidable) amounts of foreign DNA (like those from the mouse) into those receiving treatment. Even worse would be the cells themselves creating a proliferation of non-self-organisms that continue to replicate in the body causing unknown future ramifications, like allergies and auto-immune disorders or a threat to natural immunity.

The idea of proliferating antibodies may seem like a better solution than previous vaccines, as the attempt is to administer only the disease-fighting B cells into a person that is supposed to target specific antigens. But, while the theory and scientific jargon sound plausible, the material they are harvesting does NOT perform the same as our own antibodies and SUPRESSES our own immunity. As we have seen before, the presence of antibodies does not keep someone from experiencing sickness and disease, how can we think that cloning and administration of antibodies will be the answer to disease in the world? We must keep in mind that the blood, where our immune system lies, is a living, active, and highly complicated process. Even if we could create antibodies against specific antigens, there is no way we could do this effectively for all pathogens we will encounter. (or possibly create?)

### What We Do Know About Monoclonal Antibodies

- As in the past, the creation of these mAbs requires proliferation of disease (or disease-causing antigens).
- People who have been shown (in their blood) to have antigen-specific antibodies, still can get (and often do) the same exact disease that they have been "immunized" against.

- Exposure to other viruses (foreign and diseased matter) is inevitable.
- It's likely that mAbs do, and will, contribute to and cause: allergic reactions, decreased/suppressed immunity, auto-immune disorders, viral disease and cancer.
- The SARS CoV-2 Monoclonal antibody vaccines were claimed to be effective against COVID, but there is now much overwhelming evidence that these vaccines not only caused COVID, but a huge array of devastating complications far worse than anything any unvaccinated people were experiencing including: SARS, Heart attacks, Nervous and CNS damage, loss of function (physical, cognitive etc.), sudden onset diabetes, cancer and more.
- While I consider myself unqualified to make a statement on whether anyone has seen some kind of improvement of specific conditions that mAbs have been prescribed to treat, I think it's worth noting that in no case does such treatment prevent or cure any of the underlying conditions. From targeted cancer treatment to reduction of inflammation, in nearly (if not every) case, the mAbs chief mechanism of action serves to suppress the immune system's alarm response: IE Histamine/ inflammatory response etc. set off (in the first place) by the trauma of an over-abundance of viral particles, toxins and other antigens as well as vaccines and drugs.

Dr. Patrick Soon-Shiong brings up the point, in his interview with Tucker Carlson, that this hyper focus on antibody-producing drugs/vaccines has diminished the body's ability to efficiently locate and destroy harmful viruses (foreign invaders) and destroy them due to the suppression of the Killer T cells of the immune system. While he points out the sad reality that we are seeing serious diseases and cancers in the very young in a way that was unheard of before (thanks to our COVID injections), he has had success helping people heal from what would've been life-threatening cancer simply by empowering the body to re-activate their T-cells and attack the foreign invaders through his Bio shield injections.

The body's immune system is a highly complex and delicate system, capable of extinguishing nearly every threat to the body if given the chance to do so. It ought to be supported not suppressed.

In our pursuit and obsession of antibody creation and injection we are, once again, doing more harm than good. While thinking we can create better immunity by forcing change, we are failing to realize that we are creating dis-regulation and undermining the necessary balance of our body's systems. Also, we are shedding the informational patterns of disease to our fellow man at a never-ending rate. The only thing that seems more devastating is gene-altering "therapies" that could permanently defile and alter our humanity.

# CHAPTER 9

## 1ST DO NO HARM

Whether this phrase originated with Hippocrates, Thomas Sydenham or is simply a phrase, the ideas of which are so famous, it doesn't really matter who said it, all well-meaning (or right-hearted) physicians and health care workers, should live by its essence. Shouldn't they? Yet, the reality of the medical establishment fails to follow such advice. It is estimated that approximately 250,000 deaths in the United States each year are due to medical errors, which means it is the third highest cause of death in the country. And those numbers are likely much smaller than the reality.

One could certainly argue that no treatment at all may be desirable over going to the doctor for most ailments. I believe this is the reason why men who feared doctors, throughout history, seemed, in their time, to be of better health and live longer than the average person. This included kings from the Middle Ages who, rightfully, mistrusted the medical profession altogether.

But now, we live in an era that is supposed to be at its peak, both in knowledge and understanding and practice, as well as the best medical advancements, tools, devices and skill, that one could hope for. Yet, it would seem, rather that we are caught in a sort of perpetual dark ages when it comes to practices that should have been long dispelled. Also, the lack of understanding even in basic areas as real nutrition and natural plant "biologicals" puts the medical establishment at a real disadvantage in disease prevention and treatment. Diagnosing certainly fails to address root issues in many cases, if issues are even properly diagnosed at all.

At the very least, this area of injecting toxoids, chemicals, biologicals or adjuvants as well as any other material foreign or even natural into the bloodstream or body of a person, should be done away with as it is neither advantageous nor safe.

Yet, while safety is held in such high esteem so often by nurses and practitioners, and stringent rules about cleanliness and proper procedures are upheld by most (or all) hospitals, all safety, and even common sense seem to be thrown to the wind when it comes to vaccines.

## Informed Consent?

What the insert of a Hep. B Vaccine tells practitioners is their duty to do:

"PATIENT COUNSELING INFORMATION

Information for Vaccine Recipients and Parents/Guardians

• Inform the patient, parent or guardian of the potential benefits and risks associated with vaccination, as well as the importance of completing the immunization series.

• Question the vaccine recipient, parent or guardian about the occurrence of any symptoms and/or signs of adverse reaction after a previous dose of hepatitis B vaccine.
• Tell the patient, parent or guardian to report adverse events to the physician or clinic where the vaccine was administered.
• Prior to vaccination, give the patient, parent or guardian the Vaccine Information Statements which are required by the National Vaccine Injury Act of 1986. The materials are available free of charge at the Centers for Disease Control and Prevention (CDC) website (www.cdc.gov/vaccines).
• Tell the patient, parent or guardian that the United States Department of Health and Human Services has established a Vaccine Adverse Event Reporting System (VAERS) to accept all reports of suspected adverse events after the administration of any vaccine, including but not limited to the reporting of events by the National Childhood Vaccine Injury Act of 1986. The VAERS toll-free number is 1-800-822-7967. Reporting forms may also be obtained at the VAERS website at (www.vaers.hhs.gov)."

How many doctors do you know that ever discussed any of these items before, during and after vaccinating a patient? I certainly don't know of any. Of course it does not work well, because vaccines are very, Not Safe, and any symptoms following, and even reported to a physician, is simply written off as a coincidence or ignored.

While it is true that most practitioners are unaware of the actual ingredients or deadly consequences associated with vaccines, it is a poor excuse to continue a harmful practice that you (or they), as the doctor or practitioner bear responsibility for. It is also true, that if you web search any topics associated with vaccines and the related info about their respective diseases, you will not find the truth.

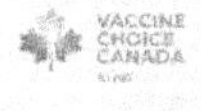


**RISK OF DEATH**
**VACCINES VS. DISEASES**

| DISEASE | RISK OF DISEASE DEATH | RISK OF VACCINE DEATH |
|---|---|---|
| Diphtheria | < 1/42,509,839 | < 1 / 76,341 |
| Tetanus | <1/1,506,184 | < 1 / 76,341 |
| Pertussis | < 1/2,346,718 | < 1 / 76,341 |
| Polio | < 1 / 1 trillion | < 1 / 214,973 |
| Measles | < 1 / 106,506,429 | < 1 / 108,666 |
| Mumps | < 1 / 40,371,594 | < 1 / 108,666 |
| Rubella | 0 to negligible | < 1 / 108,666 |
| Varicella | < 1 / 32,331,860 | < 1 / 202,398 |
| Hepatitis A | < 1 / 1,667,135 | < 1 / 72,948 |
| Hepatitis B | < 1 / 305,465 | < 1 / 96,314 |
| Hib | < 1 / 1,494,710 | < 1 / 45,966 |
| Pneumococcal | < 1 / 236,562 | < 1 / 50,056 |
| Meningococcal | < 1 / 821,925 | < 1 / 141,124 |
| Influenza | < 1 / 135,905 | < 1 / 15,702 |

**IN EVERY CASE, THE RISK OF DEATH FROM THE VACCINE EXCEEDS THE RISK OF DEATH FROM THE DISEASE**

I want to include an excerpt from Dr. Palevsky, who administered vaccines to children and families in his practice, but he had eyes to see the damage being caused right in front of his eyes. The following is his observations in his own words:

# Dr. Lawrence Palevsky

The Unvaccinated Children, "are the Healthiest Children I Have Ever Seen."

LEGISLATIVE INFORMATIONAL FORUM - To discuss Connecticut's policies on required immunizations for public school children (Tetyana Obukhanych)

“My name is Dr. Lawrence Palevsky, and I am a pediatrician, originally trained at NYU of medicine, graduated in 1987, finished my residency in Mt. Sinai Hospital in New York in 1990; did a fellowship at the Belleview hospital in the outpatient department. The first nine years of my career were spent in ERs, running an intensive care unit, working in a neo natal intensive care unit, working in-patient in the hospital, working in a clinic and then eventually, having a private practice.

In 1983, when I started medical school, I was taught vaccines were safe and they were effective and gave them, but I was not taught about any of the science around their safety or any of the studies... that were done, and it was not until 1998 that a mother came up to me and said, "Dr. Larry, Did you know there is mercury in vaccines?" and I said, "No, I did not." and as a medical student, I was trained to critically think. If you see an observation, you go after it and try to figure out if there is a question to ask.

So instead of just ignoring it, I looked further into the vaccine ingredients, and I found that there were a number of vaccines ingredients, that in animal studies were proven to be very dangerous to animals and I didn't understand why the same ingredients were actually in vaccines.

I was starting to hear stories from parents, not dozens, not hundreds but thousands of stories from parents who took a very healthy child into their doctor's office and then found that their child lost much of their health, whether it was their speech, whether it was seizures, whether it was death, whether it was asthma, allergies, eczema, whether it was autism, whether it was learning disabilities, whether it was inflammatory bowel disease, auto-immune diseases and every one of those parents were told it had nothing to do with the vaccines; every single one. And this continues today, but yet, when I look at the ingredients that are in the vaccines, I have the science to actually explain how these medical problems could be happening in these children.

Today, one child in five is learning disabled. In 1976, it was one in seventeen. One in six under age eight, one in two adolescents and one in four young adults is diagnosed with a mental, behavioral, or emotional disorder. One in twenty children under the age of five has seizures. One child in forty develops autism. The number of cases of children and adults of auto immune diseases is rising exponentially. It is one of the highest rising diseases in this country, and the vaccine ingredients, if you are willing to look into them and understand how they work when they are injected into the body, can be seen to be responsible for every single one of these cases.

So, what are these ingredients? Well, when I was in medical school, we were taught that the body has something called the blood/brain barrier. The blood brain barrier is like Fort Knox to the brain. Elements of the blood stream cannot get into the brain and those elements include drugs, viruses and bacteria, among other things in the blood.

Drug companies were very concerned about being able to develop drugs, to get the drugs into the brain and so they used something called a nanoparticle. A Nanoparticle is a very small particle bound to the drug, and they found that if they could put a nanoparticle onto a drug, they could get that drug to go into the brain, and it shows in animal studies that they were able to do this. They then were able to take an emulsifier, which is something that is good with water and fat and can dissolve in both, and if they added the emulsifier to the nanoparticle, bound to the drug, they could increase drug entry into the brain, twenty-fold. This is right out of animal studies that I found. So, you have a drug, you have a nanoparticle, and you have this emulsifier. The vaccines are constructed the same way.

You have the vaccine viruses and bacteria that are bound to a nanoparticle called aluminum, and that aluminum is a nanoparticle and by definition, a nanoparticle has the potential to enter the brain. Most vaccines also contain polysorbate 80 or sorbitol. Both of those compounds are emulsifiers. Emulsifiers bind very tightly to the nanoparticle aluminum which is bound very tightly to the vaccine antigens.

This raises a question. If the vaccine model is the same model as the [animal] model that the drug companies are using to enhance the delivery of drugs into the brain, is it possible that vaccine ingredients are making their way into the brains of our children? That could explain why so many parents are watching their kids deteriorate after vaccinations, even though the doctors, the media and the government say, "absolutely no connection" even though the science suggests that there is.

You cannot find a single study in the literature that addresses whether the injection of aluminum into the body penetrates the brain, whether any vaccine ingredients enter the brain, and whether poly sorbate 80 enhances the delivery of any of those ingredients into the brain and when I could not find those studies, I was concerned, because I am told, you're told, vaccines are safe; evaluated and very, very distinctly tested for safety but yet you cannot find a study that says, "Does aluminum stay in/ get into the brain of children?"

Does aluminum take other vaccine ingredients into the brain that don't belong in the brain because when ingredients get across the blood/brain barrier that don't belong in the brain, they cause inflammation and inflammation is what we see in one in five children with learning disabilities and one in forty with autism and all you have to do is ask the guidance counselors and if you get honest pediatricians who are telling you what they are seeing in their practice. They are seeing kids, one after another, with more and more brain disorders.

Now as a medical doctor who was taught to think, I then went into the literature and said, "Are proper science studies done; safety studies, where you take a vaccine and you inject it into a hundred kids and then you give a hundred kids a saline placebo; meaning it's inert." No study exists to actually evaluate the safety of a vaccine compared to a placebo group; none.

With vaccine safety, when vaccines were studied, the maximum amount of days vaccines are studied are up to ten days to two weeks and unfortunately, the vaccine manufacturers pre-select what side effects they will allow to be associated with the vaccines. So, if a child has a vaccine reaction that is associated with a vaccine, the vaccine manufacturers will decide whether or not it should or should not be associated with a vaccine, and the public knows this and they are learning it more and more.

So, if your child develops seizures five months after a vaccine, your child is told by a doctor that it had nothing to do with the vaccine. But that is not true, because there are no studies to prove it. There is opinion, but there has never been a study really addressing whether a vaccination at two months or even nine hours of age could be related to an event that happened months or even years later, and yet, we have some of the sickest children in our country. In New York, we lost the religious exemption on June 13 because the unvaccinated children with a religious exemption were blamed for a measles outbreak.

When I met with representatives in New York, I told them that there is no study to prove that unvaccinated children have ever been proven to start an epidemic and he was surprised. And he said, "I will vote against removing the religious exemption if I can't find a study like you say." He could not find a study but he voted to repeal the religious exemption anyway.

Because there are no studies, there are no studies proving that unvaccinated children are responsible. There is consensus and here is why there is consensus: We are taught that vaccines stop the children from carrying the germs that we are vaccinating against. And study after study shows that children who are vaccinated can still carry the germ despite having received the vaccine! So, the vaccinated are still capable of spreading disease but the unvaccinated are being unfairly blamed because of a consensus opinion, but not true science.

To repeat; no study, no science has ever proven that vaccines eliminate the existence of the organism in your body. If anything, science is showing that vaccines cause the organisms to mutate and there are plenty of articles showing that strains are replaced by new strains after vaccinations, similarly to the way antibiotics are bringing about new strains of bacteria because of the overuse of antibiotics.

So why are we blaming the unvaccinated children? No study has ever been done in this country, appropriate to address the health outcomes of children who are vaccinated vs. the children who are unvaccinated. I have been seeing families in my practice for over twenty years that have opted out of vaccinations. They are the healthiest children I have ever seen.

I have families who have older children who have been vaccinated, middle children who have been partially vaccinated and then younger children who have not been vaccinated at all, and those families are rising in number and they see the difference between the health outcomes of their younger children who are rarely sick vs. their older children who, are getting IEPs in schools, needing medications, ERs, and constant health issues and all I get when I hear that, when I state something like that is, "Well that is just anecdotal." Well, it is anecdotal if you see it a couple of times but it is not anecdotal when you see it for over 20 yrs. and when you speak to parents, and when you speak to teachers and when you speak to guidance counselors and when I speak to pediatricians who are too afraid to come out in public.

There is pressure to ostracize the families who know the science and know the lack of science that is available. There is a lot of consensuses and when I think about the subject of vaccination, I want to ensure that if we are going to prevent infectious diseases in children that we don't create something worse in its place.

Unfortunately, we are dealing with a lot of beliefs instead of actual science and beliefs go a long way. I took the oath of first, do no harm but when I look into the science and I don't see long-term studies and I see only short-term studies, up to four to ten days, where the side effects are manipulated by the manufacturers (who are the only ones doing the study on the vaccines). And when I see no placebo groups and I see no studies of the single ingredients or the combined ingredients; and I see the science, the biochemistry of the ingredients in animal studies, where animals were given the aluminum and are found to have motor delays and behavioral problems, which is a great deal of what we are seeing in children today. I say, are we first doing no harm? And so, first doing no harm means the precautionary principle. And more and more parents are understanding the dangers of vaccines and that is why we are seeing such pressure to mandate vaccines, because more of the science is coming out.

In order to create herd immunity, you have to be able to prove that children who are vaccinated are immune, and the sad part about that is that whenever you vaccinate a population of children, you are always going to have a population that doesn't develop any antibodies at all. The estimates of that are about 10 percent, that vaccines will fail in 10 percent of the population.

Vaccination, no antibody production.

But the next group is even more suspicious because when you vaccinate, and you do produce an antibody, **there is science to show that the presence of an antibody doesn't guarantee immunity either**. We don't know the percentage of children who get a vaccine, develop an antibody but aren't immune at all. We assume that if we vaccinate, we are getting protection. We assume that if we vaccinate we are stopping the spread of disease. Those are assumptions that have never been solidified in science and I am happy to offer more explanations during the Q and A. I wouldn't say that if I didn't have the science to prove it.

The parents that I work with in New York, that I see around the country are very concerned that their rights are being taken away, that their knowledge about the science is being pushed away by an agenda that only says, "unvaccinated children are a problem."

Just to wrap up, in New York when we had the measles outbreak, I am sorry, in California when they had a measles outbreak; there were one-hundred and ninety-four cases. Of the one-hundred and ninety-four cases, seventy-three cases were due to the actual virus in the vaccine itself. Seventy-three cases; 38%. Seventy-three cases were due to the measles virus, [in the vaccine] causing measles. All the literature states that measles virus infection is not true measles and should not be counted as a health threat. That means that only one-hundred, twenty-one kids developed measles. One-hundred twenty-one people.

New York State did not do the proper testing that is given by the CDC to test every child to see if the children had measles strain, wild type measles or a mutated measles. There are cases around the country and around the world, where in a 95 to 98% vaccinated population, they had measles outbreaks because they found mutated viruses.

As I said before, there are cases where the virus mutates. There are strain replacements. New York State did not do the proper testing of the 1000 plus young children and adults who came down with measles. They wrote a little blurb on the CDC website of the two wild viruses that were responsible for the measles outbreak but we in New York know that the testing was not done. Forty-two hundred kids on Long Island, who had the religious exemption and were not vaccinated and there was not one case of measles on Long Island.

Thank you."

The video cannot be viewed, because it has since been removed. I do wish people could watch it in its original format. Here, is a transcript of a doctor who tried his utmost to do the right thing. He took his oath and his profession seriously, as one who has true compassion and takes responsibility for his patients. Many, like him, have risen up to try and be a voice against the damaging effects of vaccines. A few of them still persist. Most are gone, never to be heard from again. This is an evil we cannot allow to continue. We also must keep some of these truths from the past, for if we allow this history to disintegrate, we will, as the saying goes, be "condemned to repeat it."

# RFK on the MMR

From "Defending" Children's Health to Destroying It: Robert F. Kennedy Jr. Now Recommends MMR Vaccine After Years of Condemning It

At the time of writing this, this post can still be found at the above address.

Robert F. Kennedy Jr., Trump's Secretary of Health and Human Services (HHS), published an opinion piece yesterday on Fox News about the current "measles outbreak." He wrote: "MMR vaccine is crucial to avoiding potentially deadly disease. Vaccines not only protect individual children from measles, but also contribute to community immunity, protecting those who are unable to be vaccinated due to medical reasons." Here is what Robert F. Kennedy wrote about the fraudulent MMR vaccine by Merck back in 2019: "If you multiply the known adverse events from the MMR by 100, you get 44,500 deaths and 8,900,000 injuries making the measles vaccine far worse than measles." The MMR is a 3-vaccine combo vaccine for measles, mumps, and rubella. There is no actual "measles vaccine." It has been established that the MMR vaccine is linked to increased levels of autism in children.

Dr. Andrew Wakefield, the poster-boy for Big Pharma who like to state the claim that the "MMR vaccine causes autism has been scientifically debunked," was the first one to go public with his concerns about the MMR vaccine and its link to autism.

In 2014, Dr. Wakefield was exonerated when a CDC scientist who worked on the original study that the CDC says proves the MMR vaccine does not cause autism, confessed to Brian Hooker in a phone call that they had fabricated the study, and that his conscience continually bothered him about the fraudulent study. The scientist's name is Dr. William Thompson. Dr. Andrew Wakefield produced a video about his admission of guilt. It is hard to find on the Internet these days, but we have a copy." "we" meaning, those at *Health Impact News*."

The video he is referring to is surely the VAXXED Documentary. The series contains vital information about the realities of vaccine damage (undeniable). It is true that the series is hard to find: The vaxxedthemovie.com website has been hacked (now re-directs to an HVAC Co), the video has been taken off You Tube (for "violating standards") and the only place you can find it to view are websites like, Children's Health Defense or Rumble.

When RFK became the secretary of the HHS, some of us thought it was too good to be true. Demanding that poison stop becoming FDA approved and that doctors stop forcibly injecting toxins into our children etc. etc.

Regarding our current leaders (in 2025), I must say, particularly in vaccination exemption rights and exposure of the evils of both the diet food industry and medical malpractice, RFK was THE man for the job. He was there, when the VAXXED bus put thousands of names of vaccine injured children, women and adults who suffered some of the worst reactions imaginable including death. He heard their stories, and multitudes of others; he vowed to represent these children and their families in court and in the political arena, until justice was served. He awed and inspired the masses (myself included) with his beautiful words on freedom, health and justice. But what I am finding more and more is that, not only has he never come right out and stated he was "anti-vaccine," he also seems to advocate that he was never anti-vaccine-mandate. Instead, his emphasis (the part he's wanted us to hear) is that he's for "vaccine safety," which really is a misnomer, as there is NO SUCH THING as a Safe Vaccine. I know many are still hopeful that RFK has a "PLAN." I hope so (and that it is a good plan) but regardless, this is NOT an area I will continue to allow government officials to handle without taking personal responsibility for what I know to be true.

Most recently, in an article by *USA Today* It has been reported that RFK has fired 17 CDC employees that advise the country on the safety of vaccines and is replacing them with new members.

"Today we are prioritizing the restoration of public trust above any specific pro- or anti-vaccine agenda," Kennedy Jr. says. Note how he affirms the plan to rebuild the people's trust over abolishing vaccines. While I am not disregarding positive progress towards transparency, transparency is something that may become elusive far too quickly, especially in a world steeped in the innovative abilities of AI technology. What I am advocating for is to keep awake and be careful to accept any narrative that creates some new reason to accept vaccines, no matter who is advocating for it.

The most recent news (as of June 26, 2025), is that the new 8 member committee appointed by RFK just voted to recommend a new RSV Vaccine for Infants. This is a monoclonal antibody vaccine created by Merck. So, we are already seeing an addition, not reduction, in the number of vaccines being recommended by the HHR.

What if we are now looking upon a new, open door for more vehicles of mass destruction to be widely implemented? I believe there is a spiritual agenda behind the scenes that continues because even those who mean well have judgement still clouded by wrong ideologies in the world of health. Millions upon millions more could be damaged, and their stories stifled, and the blame shifted and the narrative controlled, until what should have been obvious becomes a new, twisted narrative. There won't be a better time to stand up and fight this issue. If no one does, we may lose the opportunity altogether, and the agenda of vaccinating the entire world will happen sooner than we might think, and may lead to an unimaginable, worldwide disaster there will be no coming back from.

# CHAPTER 10

## DON'T FEAR THEM.

I still remember the days when I used to feel bad about declining vaccines. I didn't want to be seen as a negligent or uncooperative parent. Furthermore, I felt a certain amount of fear from the medical establishment and doctors as well as the system at large: possible government involvement, CPS, powers beyond my small self that made me feel like I needed to cooperate. I no longer feel that way. I have acquired much more information and understanding about the evils of vaccination and have also grown in my position and standing against them. As I have done so, I find that the opposition has become significantly less. Doctors don't pressure moms who are stalwart about their decisions concerning the care of their children. Those who are most ignorant and most vulnerable, I really do believe, get prayed on and pressured the hardest. When I became so firm on my convictions that I hoped a doctor would challenge me on the subject, none did.

This is not an attack on doctors or staff. Though I still dislike being a patient in hospitals, I have felt a deep gratitude for many practitioners, particularly specialists, whose care and intervention were a difference between life and death: not for me but for my last two (and particularly last) babies, who required special monitoring, interventions and even blood transfusions to keep them from severe injury and possible death.

A friend of mine shared a story of when she felt pressured by her doctor to accept a vaccine while she was pregnant. Sadly, her story is more common than those in her position usually feel.

She says, "When I was pregnant my first time in 1999-2000, I used my OB/GYN. I'd been a patient of his for ten years and I trusted him. During that pregnancy, we were advised to research the issue of vaccines. That was my first exposure to realizing they weren't safe or biblically clean. We made the decision to avoid them. But, at one of my monthly prenatal appointments, I was told I was getting a flu shot that day. I politely declined and that led to a 'polite lecture' and lots of pressure to take the shot. I'm ashamed to admit that I caved into the pressure and took that flu shot."

I don't feel the need to relay the entire episode, which, for her was quite emotional, as it would be for anyone who had felt pressured to do something that she felt violated her conscience, during a season when she and her husband were just beginning to learn of the reality of the danger of vaccines. The conflict between wanting to follow the advice of someone you have trusted for you and your baby's health, fear of how you will be perceived if you don't comply contrasted with things you know and others have shared about vaccine dangers and their ingredients, as well as your own gut feelings and cautions are all things that have caused an internal struggle for so many moms wanting to do the right thing.

This mother did observe complications with her newborn son following vaccination, which she later regretted.

"My son was born with food allergies and food sensitivities that plagued him for years. He also cried (screamed) for 10-12 hours a day for the first 3 months of his life. It was so awful. I know they call it 'colic' but looking back I now believe it was a reaction to the shot. I can't prove it but it's my gut feeling that the flu shot affected his little body."

While I wouldn't use stories like this as scientific proof that vaccines cause all these issues; the number of stories similar to this one, whose mothers looked back, later researched the adverse reactions of vaccines, noticed certain patterns in their children's behavior, started connecting dots from their own experience and others, etc. are so numerous that they should at least be acknowledged, for there are many of them.

I don't want any mom to ever have to feel fearful about deciding not to vaccinate their children. This is a main reason I felt compelled to write this book. Parents are being led to believe that waiting, spacing them out, and monitoring the effects will erase all needed concerns about vaccines. They won't.

I am sorry that there is a stigma about being "anti-vax." There shouldn't be. I will firmly proclaim my anti-vaccine stance to the end. Most things are not black and white. Disease is one of those things. Usually, I bank on the side of: all things are complicated and one size does not fit all, especially in the area of health, including diet, and a multitude of health decisions. Vaccines are NOT a "grey area." They are not "worth the risk." Their only value has ever been in producing evil. This evil is far broader and goes far deeper than we've discussed in this book. There are agendas and depopulation and sterilization goals that are wrapped into this practice, as well as the desire to create a surplus of individuals ripe for medical practice. As Dr. Mendelsohn declares, "The pediatrician indoctrinates your child from birth into a lifelong dependency on medical intervention…" and Sherri Tenpenny, "Vaccines are the backbone of the entire Pharmaceutical Industry. If they can make these children sick from a very early age, they become customers for life."

There is not only the spirit of deception, but of control, manipulation and destruction that is rooted in something far more sinister, and far more spiritual then most people talk about. There is much more history about the evils of vaccines than can be found in this book. There are several more I mention in the appendices with history I haven't even used in this book, like: ***Dissolving Illusions*** by Suzanne Humphries and Roman Bystrianyk, which is all about the forgotten history of disease and vaccines, as well as several other references mentioned.

Let history be the teacher. Let the stories of innumerable amounts of damage from children harmed by this perpetual practice be your informers. Don't let the damage continue. Don't let the persecutors get to you. Doctors don't realize what they're doing when they pressure parents into vaccinating their children. In some cases, it should be obvious that the spirit behind their insistence is an evil, or at least unethical one. There IS an evil behind the perpetuation of vaccination. Do NOT be intimidated by evil. Stand up to evil. Stand up to bullies, or they will bully someone else. Evil only has power over individuals who allow it to have power. All who know the extent to which vaccines have caused hurt and damage understand why it is evil. This is not just a "better choice" or debatable practice. There are many debatable practices. There is a particular evil present when it comes to vaccines, and I believe this evil is going to get worse. You are not making a bad decision for deciding not to vaccinate. You are a good parent. Don't let ANYONE tell you different.

The people who should be afraid are the ones involved in and allowing the damage to continue. Those who are good-willed, but ignorant on the matter, will change their opinion when presented with the facts.

It may be a big dream, but it would surely be wonderful if this evil were fully eradicated. If enough people stood up against this administration, it would lose its power, even if it remained in practice. And we would have enough "normal" healthy people to show that vaccination is NOT THE WAY to be healthy.

## Come Out of the Dark Ages

"Declaring themselves to be wise, they became fools." Rom. 1:22

If there is a root definition of an era of "Dark Ages" it would be the falling away or forgetting of what came before. While many histories may be lost to the world, if we had at least adhered to the pages of the Bible and its ideas on health, we surely could not have descended so deeply into delusion. The book of Leviticus, for example, contains practices of isolation and cleansing to irradicate diseases that are actively proliferating. Perhaps if men had not become so "wise" as to decide that these ancient texts were irrelevant to their "enlightened age" or if people had sought their maker for answers in their sickness and not forgot some of the most basic principles of life and cleanliness, much pain and disease could've been irradicated.

Instead, they looked to themselves, or in essence, men who had erroneous ideas about how to manage disease. As one example, we should have never found ourselves in a position of thinking it ridiculous to need to wash our hands, after dealing with literal, physical processes of death, to assisting with the delicate process of life. Eras of darkness are surely spiritual darkness, and, I believe, a willful ignorance that stems, most likely, from willful pride. The ideas of treatments during these eras were dark and the superstitions that held people captive to unseemly and hurtful practices were spiritual. This is not about shaming or condemning a certain era of history, but I think this is an important realization in understanding the real reason for sickness and disease in the first place. The idea of how disease develops in a human body had to first descend away from the idea of the created order into a theory of a microbial world which continually blamed the wrong culprit for the problems of life. A theory that misunderstood how or why the microbial world existed.

While we are engulfed in this "age of information" we still linger in a bit of dark ages when we embrace cult-like practices that should've been extinguished long ago. Vaccination is indeed a cult. It is a very wide-spread and now nationally accepted cult that continues to plague our medical systems. It's not neutral. It has become an administration through which the Devil can do his work: of creating as much destruction and defilement as possible and is consistent with his devices: use of greed, fear and ignorance to continue the cycle. I have always believed (or felt) that the reason people were so willing to accept this germ theory, along with its awful ramifications, is that it seemed to give people an element (or feeling) of control over the disease process. Including the idea that, through the "power of vaccination," we could "irradicate diseases," as though we are making some great, revolutionary, human achievement. Acts as humble as taking care of our own living space, praying to God for healing, being willing change, serve each other, and admit if we are wrong, had no place in this "new, revolutionary era over disease."

I could say a lot in this section, indeed, even point out that the whole history of the inception of vaccines throughout its use has been built on a kingdom in opposition to truth and light in every way.

In very short summary: Vaccination has been an evil that began with lies and empty promises and compromise and was built on greed, deception, sacrifice and defilement, and propelled by position, prestige and pride, and perpetuated by fear, deceit and darkness. It's time that the real history of vaccination be brought into the light!

## The Story of The People Vs David and Collett Stephan

I want to end this chapter with a story about a family, who is a friend of a friend, who lost their son, tragically due to a mistake made by the medical team who took him to the hospital. While they didn't understand it, at the time, they began unraveling the mysteries that led up to the truth about their son's death and uncovered secrets and behind-the-scenes practices that had been ongoing but well-hidden in the medical establishment and court system in Canada.

The ruthless and cruel way the medical establishment portrayed them to the public eye, which led the heart-broken mom to nearly commit suicide, was all to cover their tracks, and influence other families to vaccinate their children.

Though heart wrenching, the best outcome of this story was not just in the discovering of truth to prevent what they went through from happening to others, but the journey of going from a place of fear and confusion to empowerment and fearlessness, as the truth they uncovered made them realize just how corrupt the system in this area of healthcare truly is, and that those who use their voice or power to intimidate others are nothing more than bullies.

This is just one of many stories I could mention about families who have been unfairly and ruthlessly slandered to deflect blame from the medical world unto the parents of these poor children. The Truth I believe this story conveys is that those who have nothing to hide have a force on their side greater than those willing to compromise and perpetuate evil, for the sake of gain or any other reason. If you need encouragement to fearlessly take a stand against the evil or intimidation found in certain medical circles, I invite you to check out their story.

Those who are trying to hide the reality of the damage far too often found in mainstream medical practices would like everyone involved to feel as though they are alone in their opinions and suffering, and that it is their fault. I hope that this book will help people to realize that they are far from alone.

In conclusion, I would greatly encourage you to not leave this issue in the hands of government officials. Take responsibility for your own health and your children's health, and tell your doctor, NO! Hand them one of these books. If you are a physician, please take time out of your busy schedule, to truly research this topic (apart from the collective medical narrative), because you will be held responsible for the damage done to those you prescribe vaccines for.

This is the reason I created this book in the first place: to inform people; to give people a tool (a package of information) to empower them to make the best decisions possible for their children and families; to get them started on the journey of discovering the truth in this area.
(link to story in Appendix sect: Videos, Posts & FB Links)

Note: I realize many may be reading this as a hard copy. **To view the stories and follow the links, I suggest taking a photo on your phone and then copying and pasting into your browser.**

Also, I must recognize that not all links may be viewable and it is possible some of them may have been removed since the time of this publication.

I wish you blessings on this journey and thank you for taking the time to read and/or share the material in this book.

Sincerely,

Rachel Banura

# Appendices and More Information:

Disclaimer: While great care has been taken to preserve the external links, due to the ever-changing nature of the internet, there can be no guarantee that the information and web pages still exist or that the links will appropriately deliver to the proper address.

## Informed Consent

The First Section I want to include is Resources and Information about **Informed Consent and Your Rights to Oppose Vaccines** for you or your child. Many of these will be Links or Addresses to Websites or materials, as it would take far too much space to include all of them here.

Most of the resources in this section I will be borrowing from Sarah Peterson and her Path to Freedom Website: https://www.skool.com/pathtofreedom/classroom

**In the Classroom Section**

She has compiled a great many resources and information about Vaccines, which would overfill a book 10 times this size. If you are looking for more information, and an abundance of info in this area, I would encourage you to check out her FB page and Website. It is $5/ mo. to join her Path to Freedom community, and it is very worth it, for the wealth of information there: from Homesteading to Vaccines.

The following is taken from The AAPS Opposes Federal Vaccine Mandates: Find the original post, here: https://aapsonline.org/measles-outbreak-and-federal-vaccine-mandates/

**General Info**

Informed Consent: Safeguarding Autonomy and Medical Freedom In the context of vaccination; informed consent is a critical ethical and legal principle that ensures individuals have the right to make informed decisions about their health. It requires healthcare providers to provide comprehensive and transparent information about vaccines, including their benefits, potential risks, and alternatives. Informed consent respects the fundamental principle of individual autonomy, granting individuals the right to make decisions about their own bodies. By providing comprehensive information on vaccines, including their efficacy, safety, potential side effects, and alternative options, healthcare providers empower individuals to make informed choices based on their own values, beliefs, and unique circumstances. This ensures that vaccination decisions are made voluntarily, without coercion or undue external influence.

**Transparency and Trust:** Informed consent in vaccination fosters trust between healthcare providers and individuals. When healthcare professionals openly discuss the benefits and risks of vaccines, they demonstrate a commitment to transparency and honesty. This transparency helps provide accurate information and addresses concerns.

**Risk-Benefit Assessment**: Informed consent allows individuals to assess the risks and benefits of vaccination, enabling them to make decisions based on their personal circumstances. It acknowledges that different individuals may have varying levels of risk tolerance or unique medical conditions that could affect the appropriateness of certain vaccines. By understanding the potential benefits and risks, individuals can weigh the overall risk benefit profile of vaccination and make informed choices that align with their health priorities. Protection Against Coercion and Infringement of Rights: Providing informed consent before vaccination safeguards individuals from coercion and potential infringement of their rights. It ensures that vaccination decisions are made voluntarily and without undue pressure. Informed consent acts as a safeguard against mandatory vaccination policies that may violate individual rights or personal beliefs. Respecting informed consent preserves the autonomy and freedom of individuals, allowing them to maintain control over their bodies and healthcare choices. Informed consent before vaccination is a fundamental principle that upholds individual autonomy, fosters trust in healthcare, protects against coercion, and promotes public health. By providing comprehensive and transparent information, healthcare providers empower individuals to make decisions based on their own values and circumstances. Informed consent strengthens the partnership between healthcare providers and patients, ensuring that vaccination decisions are made voluntarily and respect individual rights. Embracing informed consent in vaccination reinforces the importance of autonomy, trust, and collective well-being in our healthcare systems.

Unfortunately, in today's society, many doctors (especially pediatricians) do not provide informed consent. Parents are handed a quick print-out of which vaccines their child will be receiving and normally are given just a few minutes to go over the information. The information given is provided by a 3rd party company that contracts out with doctor's offices, they do not come from the vaccine manufacturer. If the parent doesn't agree to vaccinate, even if it's due to not having enough time to consider the information they've been given, they can risk having their doctor's office let them go as a patient. That is NOT informed consent.

The Moral Right to Conscientious, Philosophical and Personal Belief Exemption to Vaccination

https://www.nvic.org/NVIC/media/LegacySite/pdf/downloads/the-moral-right-to-conscientious-vaccine-exemption.pdf

Children's Health Defense: What Every Parent Should Know

https://childrenshealthdefense.org/protecting-our-future/facts-you-can-use/i-wish-id-known/

https://childrenshealthdefense.org/protecting-our-future/facts-you-can-use/10-facts-every-parent-needs-to-know-about-vaccinations/

Info On Right to Refuse and Connected Bills

https://childrenshealthdefense.org/community/right-to-refuse-health-freedom-bills/

https://righttorefuse.org/

Info on Measles from the National Vaccine Information Center

https://www.nvic.org/disease-vaccine/measles

## About Compensation Programs

### National Vaccine Injury Act

The **National Vaccine Injury Act (NVICA)**, enacted in **1986**, was created to address concerns about vaccine safety, compensate individuals injured by vaccines, and protect vaccine manufacturers from excessive liability lawsuits.

**Key Points of the Act:**

1. **Created the National Vaccine Injury Compensation Program (VICP)** – This is a **no-fault compensation program** that provides financial compensation to individuals who suffer injuries or adverse reactions from vaccines covered under the program.

2. **Established the Vaccine Adverse Event Reporting System (VAERS)** – A national system where healthcare providers, manufacturers, and the public can report vaccine-related injuries or adverse effects.
3. **Provided Liability Protections for Vaccine Manufacturers** – It shielded manufacturers from lawsuits related to vaccine injuries, encouraging the continued production of vaccines while still ensuring a compensation pathway for those injured.
4. **Created the Vaccine Injury Table** – A list of recognized vaccine injuries that qualify for compensation without the burden of proving causation.
5. **Mandated Informed Consent and Vaccine Information Statements (VIS)** – Requires healthcare providers to give patients standardized information about vaccine benefits and potential risks.

**Why Was It Passed?**

In the **1980s**, lawsuits against vaccine manufacturers increased due to claims of vaccine injuries, particularly from the **DTP (Diphtheria, Tetanus, and Pertussis) vaccine**. This led to some manufacturers **stopping vaccine production**, creating concerns about shortages. The NVICA aimed to balance public health needs with legal protections.

**How Does It Work Today?**

- People who believe they have suffered a vaccine injury can file a claim with the **VICP**, which is managed by the **U.S. Court of Federal Claims**.
- If a case qualifies, compensation covers medical costs, lost earnings, and pain/suffering.
- Claims are funded through a **$0.75 excise tax per vaccine dose**, not by pharmaceutical companies directly.

The **NVICA does not cover COVID-19 vaccines**, which currently fall under the separate **Countermeasures Injury Compensation Program (CICP)**.

The **National Vaccine Injury Compensation Act (NVICA)** has several flaws and limitations that have been widely debated. Here are the key criticisms:

**1. Compensation Process is Lengthy and Complex**

- The **National Vaccine Injury Compensation Program (VICP)** was meant to be a **quick and fair** alternative to lawsuits, but many claimants **wait years** for resolution.
- Petitioners often **face significant legal hurdles**, requiring expert medical testimony to prove injury causation, even for cases that seem straightforward.
- The process can be costly for claimants, despite the program covering some legal fees.

**2. Vaccine Manufacturers Are Shielded from Liability**

- One of the main criticisms is that **vaccine manufacturers cannot be sued for design defects** in court, even if evidence suggests they knew of risks.

- This means there is **no incentive for pharmaceutical companies to improve vaccine safety**, as they are **not held financially accountable** for injuries.

**3. The Burden of Proof is on the Injured Party**

- Even though the program is called "no-fault," individuals still **must prove their injury was caused by the vaccine.**
- The **Vaccine Injury Table** lists certain injuries that automatically qualify for compensation, but many legitimate injuries **are not listed**, making claims harder to win.
- If an injury is not on the table, the petitioner must **go through a rigorous legal battle** to prove causation.

**4. Many Legitimate Cases Are Denied**

- The **U.S. Court of Federal Claims (a.k.a. "Vaccine Court")** often **rejects claims**, even when medical evidence strongly suggests a vaccine-related injury.
- Some injuries occur **after a vaccine but outside the official time frame** for compensation, leaving many without financial help.

**5. Low Compensation Payouts**

- Even if a petitioner **wins their case**, the compensation can be **much lower** than what would be awarded in a civil lawsuit.
- The **pain and suffering cap** is only **$250,000**, which is far lower than what traditional courts might award for permanent disability.

**6. Limited Public Awareness**

- Many people **do not know** about the VICP and its process.
- Physicians often **fail to inform patients** about the program, and there is little public education about vaccine injuries and legal rights.

**7. Does Not Cover COVID-19 Vaccine Injuries**

- **COVID-19 vaccines are not covered** under VICP but instead fall under the **Countermeasures Injury Compensation Program (CICP)**, which is even harder to access.
- The **CICP has a much lower success rate** (less than 1% of claims are compensated) and **does not cover legal fees** for claimants.

**8. Lack of Transparency in VAERS Reporting**

- While the Vaccine Adverse Event Reporting System (VAERS) is part of NVICA, it is **passive and underreported**.
- Many doctors do **not file reports**, and injuries are dismissed as "coincidental" without proper investigation.
- VAERS data is often used to **debunk injury claims** rather than as a tool for improving vaccine safety.

**9. Conflict of Interest Concerns**

- The **U.S. Department of Health and Human Services (HHS)** oversees the VICP, but it is also responsible for **promoting and recommending vaccines**—creating a **conflict of interest**.

- Judges ruling on cases (Special Masters) **are not independent**; they work within the **same system designed to protect manufacturers**.

**10. Limited Scope of Covered Vaccines**

- Not all vaccines are covered by the VICP. New vaccines must be **added through legislation**, which means some injuries from newer vaccines **do not qualify** for compensation.

---

**Conclusion: A System That Favors Industry Over Individuals**

The NVICA was created to **balance public health and vaccine safety**, but in practice, it often **favors manufacturers and the government** over injured individuals. Many feel the program is **slow, unfair, and underfunded**, making it **difficult for victims to receive justice**.

## Vaccine Exemptions and Waivers

While many doctors and offices as well as schools, provide waivers that you can sign, and often will do so with a simple request, it may be necessary to request or create a religious exemption to refuse vaccinations. Most states still accept religious exemptions. Many accept medical exemptions, but these are usually harder to procure and require a medical doctor's signature. Few states accept Personal or Philosophical exemptions.

Note: In MI (where we live) as of 2024, parents are required to "receive education" from their county Health Dept. before acquiring a non-medical waiver form through their Health Dept. See link for table.
https://worldpopulationreview.com/state-rankings/vaccine-exemptions-by-state#title

Note from Author: While it is my personal desire to see vaccines becoming a thing of the past and eliminated completely, (and on medical/ scientific grounds. Not personal.) I want to offer any helpful information I can to empower others to avoid vaccination in our present culture. There have been many attempts to remove the religious exemption, which I'm hoping does not happen anytime soon, although as of 2024, they are already making it more difficult.
The Following are some recommendations and examples for creating and submitting a religious exemption, but you are free to create your own version for religious exemption purposes.

## Guide to Writing Religious Exemption Requests to CV-19 Vaccines:

U.S. colleges/universities and some employers are starting to require COVID-19 vaccination for enrollment/employment. While medical exemptions must be supported by a letter from a medical professional, religious exemptions do not require the support or endorsement of an official clergy or recognized religious leader. Instead, it requires that the person seeking exemption explain why his/her "sincerely held religious beliefs" prevent him/her from accepting the university's/school's/employer's requirement of vaccination.

Some universities/schools and employers will provide a specific document to fill out if you are requesting an exemption. Other times, you will need to submit your own letter. In either event, you can use this document as a general guide to help you think about and personalize your own request for a religious exemption. Please note that your request should not simply use a prepared template you find on the internet without revision. For religious exemptions to be successful, they must be unique to your own religious experience and beliefs – you must personalize the form so that it is personal to your own situation.

**Please also note: This document is not intended to provide legal advice.** It is instead a general set of suggestions or guidelines to have you thinking about how to express in writing your own sincerely held religious beliefs against vaccinating with these experimental CV-19 vaccines.

**POINTS TO REVIEW/KNOW BEFORE YOU START:**

1. A request for a religious exemption must be about religion. It is not about personal or philosophical beliefs, medical reasons for not wanting the vaccine, or legal objections to vaccine mandates. While you might be submitting other objections to taking these vaccines, do not merge those objections with your request for religious exemption.

2. The law does not require you to be a member of an organized religion, or any religion at all. However, while this is NOT required, if you are able to acquire a letter from a cleric attesting to your personal sincerity and/or your devotion to

your faith and include it with your own letter, DO IT. If you can get several letters, that is even better. It is helpful to include a history of how this person knows you and your family. A one-page letter is fine. (NEVER join a "phony" church just to get a letter like this).

3. Personalize. USE YOUR OWN WORDS. This document has SOME phrasing suggestions; modify as you see fit and as it applies to your own sincerely held religious belief situation.

4. A personal religious belief means this: You are allowed to have a personal translation of the word of your God that connects to refusing vaccines. In other words, if a religious principle (that you truly believe in) translates (in your own understanding of the word of God) to refusing vaccines, then your belief fits with the definition of a legal waiver. More details/ examples on that in the following sections.

5. Most religions do not have an official stance on vaccination. That permits the employee or college student even more freedom. The broad nature of the law enables the employee or student to honestly and easily fit with law. But always remember, your claim must always circle back to a religious belief.

6. Title VII of the Civil Rights Act of 1964 is the law that prevents employers from discriminating against an employee on the basis of their religion/religious beliefs/religious practices. It applies to employees in the workplace, rather than students in a university/college situation. However, most universities/colleges recognizing their obligation to provide religious exemptions to employees also extend this exemption option to their students, since it would violate equal protection principles and discriminate against students on the basis of their religion to fail to do so.

7. Use Words to Emphasize the Religious Nature of your Exemption Request: Sacred
   - Holy
   - Worship
   - Blessed
   - Conviction
   - Faith
   - Religious Mandate
   - Translation of the word of my God/Creator
   - Unique understanding of the language of God/Creator
   - Personal understanding of God's/Creator's message to me

## PARTS OF YOUR FORM/LETTER:

### Part 1: Request for Exemption and Statement of the Law

State your request for religious exemption and briefly state/reference the law (Title VII) that allows you such an exemption and/or accommodation:

**Example:** (you must personalize, as appropriate):

*Dear [Person you must address at your school or place of employment]*

*I am writing to formally and respectfully apply for a religious exemption to the (name of organization) Covid-19 vaccination policy that requires that all employees (or students) show proof of vaccination in order to (attend in-person school or stay employed).*

*I base my request on religious grounds. I hold sincere and genuine beliefs that forbid me from accepting a COVID-19 vaccination.*

*Under Title VII of the Civil Rights Act, an employer must not discriminate against an employee on the basis of that*

> *employee's sincerely held religious beliefs. Religious discrimination involves treating a person (an applicant or employee) unfavorably because of his or her religious beliefs. As you know, the law protects not only people who belong to traditional, organized religions, such as Buddhism, Christianity, Hinduism, Islam, and Judaism, but also others who have sincerely held religious beliefs.*

> *Note to Students: You should also cite to the school policy that allows religious exemptions for students here too. Most schools do allow them because they must allow for employees under Title VII.*

**Part 2: Request for Confidentiality**

Ask that the letter remain confidential for good reason: first and foremost so that your letter and exemption request won't be read by many eyes. Generally speaking, the fewer people charged with making the decision, the better. Additionally, there are legitimate social consequences to consider (i.e. you don't want your unvaccinated status made known so that those with preconceived prejudices/strong fears will discriminate and/or encourage others to marginalize or discriminate against you).

> *'I ask that this request for exemption be kept 100% confidential as it contains thoughts and sentiments not shared in casual conversation and deeply personal to me....'*

> *'The content of this letter is of an extremely personal nature...'*
> *'The only reason we share this with you is because the law dictates that we do...'*

> *'I ask that this be shared on an as-needed basis only; that is, only those charged with approving the exemption request should read our words.'*

**Part 3: Explain Your Sincerely Held Religious Beliefs that Prevent You from Taking the COVID-19 Vaccine:**

You need to briefly explain your religious history and religious beliefs and why these beliefs prevent you from taking the COVID-19 vaccines. No religious exemption request letter should be taken verbatim from a form/template. Since the credibility of your letter rests largely on how you express your individual personal religious belief(s), this section that defines your religious belief is essential in placing your unique signature on your description of these religious beliefs.

a. Keep in mind, this is about RELIGION, so the development of your connection to God/Creator has to be the central theme of your personal history. The information you offer must circle back to your personal relationship with God. This will create a foundation for the rest of your letter.

b. There is no reason to include traumatic events that have to do with vaccine injury. While that may be true, the reader may infer that you have medical objections to vaccinations. If you mention or highlight these events, you may cast doubt on the genuinely religious nature of your request to refuse vaccination. Stay focused.

c. While you are legally permitted to have a medical objection to vaccination and a religious objection at the same time, it is best to separate these two requests. If the school/employer has a witch hunt planned, don't buy the kindling.

d. Stick to your central objection: COVID-19 vaccination opposes *your* personal interpretation of a religious belief(s) that you hold sacred. You believe that if you were to participate in this vaccination scheme, you would be prevented from worshipping your God/Creator in the way that you see fit. If you were to take this vaccine, you would not be practicing your First Amendment Freedom of Religion. You must connect why your religious beliefs prevent you from taking these particular vaccines.

e. Possible considerations and religious objections to CV-19 mRNA and adenovirus vector vaccines: COVID-19 vaccines are the first mRNA (Pfizer/Moderna) or adenoviral vector (J & J) vaccines. These vaccines do not operate in the same way as "traditional" vaccines. Specifically, instead of using a fragment of dead virus and an adjuvant to help induce an immune response, these CV-19 vaccine products are genetic coding instructions that purport to instruct your body to produce a spike protein that is not natural to your own human genetic system. While some scientists/authorities claim that this does not alter a human's genetic structure and/or that the "vaccine" stays localized to the vaccination area (shoulder) and does not spread to the rest of the human body, other scientists and authorities disagree, and there is evidence to support their views. In any event, it is not fully known what these novel technologies are actually doing to our human DNA. The possibility of genetically altering the human body, the body created by God/Creator in His image, is something you might want to include in your reasons for not wanting to take these novel gene therapy products in particular.

f. Aborted Fetal Tissue: One can also have religious objections to vaccines based on the fact that some vaccines are created using a culture from aborted fetal tissue. Many believe that using vaccines produced from aborted fetuses shows a profound disrespect for the remains of these children. Using vaccines that exploit these deaths for profit violates the teachings of the Church. Many believe that vaccination supports abortion and consequently violates conscience. Conscience is a strong force in Christianity. However, not all vaccines are created using aborted fetal tissue. Offered in combination with other religious principles, however, it presents strong support. But these beliefs should be a component of a much larger, more comprehensive set of beliefs.

g. Use language from your applicable religious texts to support your beliefs and personal interpretation of these sacred instruction manuals – the Bible, Torah, Koran, Buddhist doctrine, etc. For example, below are some ideas that the Bible conveys that might be useful in capturing your beliefs about how COVID-19 vaccinations would violate these religious commands:

**Christian/Judeo-Christian/Biblical References:**

*The Book of Genesis states that G-d created man in His image. It is my belief that G-d knew what He was doing and the body of many needs no 'fixing' by mankind. I see vaccines as 'fixing' I cannot improve on G-d's creation. Numerous religious scriptures tell us we need to trust in G-d and His creation.*

*"Honor the Lord with your bodies." 1 Corinthians (6:20).*

*"No man can serve two masters: for either he will hate the one, and love the other; or else he will hold to the one, and despise the other. Luke (16:13)*

*Exodus 15:26 states: "If you diligently heed the voice of the Lord your God and do what is right in His sight, give ear to His Commandments and keep all His statues, I will none of the diseases on you which I brought on the Egyptians. For I am the Lord who heals you."*

*"God created us in his own image."* [Genesis 1:27]

*"So that your faith might not rest on human wisdom but on the power of God." (1 Corinthians, 2:5)*

*"Do you not know that your body is a temple of the Holy Spirit, who is in you, whom you have received from God? You are not your own. That God is in you. That he is our healer." Corinthians 6:19*

In Matthew 9:12, Jesus said: *"Those who are well do not need a physician, but the sick do."* Jesus again repeated the same in Mark 2:17. *"When Jesus heard it, he saith unto them, They that are whole have no need of the physician..."*

**Judaism/Torah References:**

You may derive your beliefs from the Torah and Judaism. Some understandings or beliefs to include might be:

*The first commandment of Jewish law is, "What does G-d expect from us?" We commit ourselves to answer that question with our own well-thought out answers. These answers are evident in all our actions, thoughts and decisions.*

*Torah prohibits we welcome foreign material into the body and this is precisely what vaccines are. I believe that it is a contradiction to fight a poison or disease that can or does enter the body with vaccination, which is disease. We believe this contradicts the teachings of the Jewish religion that mandates we keep our bodies and blood unpolluted and without contamination.*

*I consider these injections to represent defilement of the body, blood and soul and the trust we have in the healing powers of God. I believe that a body addresses disease by a good mental spirit and prayer and maintaining the purity and cleanliness of both. I do not believe that the poisons and disease of vaccines are allies in the fight against disease. I believe that our faith is our strongest support system when the body is in crisis. I believe in the healing power of prayer.*

*The Jewish religion dictates that man should not mix the blood of man and that of animals. It is well known that some vaccines are prepared using the tissue culture from animals. This directly contradicts the teachings of my faith as I see it.*

*The Book of Genesis states that G-d created man in His image. It is my belief that G-d knew what He was doing and the body of many needs no 'fixing' by mankind. I see vaccines as 'fixing' I cannot improve on G-d's creation. Numerous religious scripture tell us we need to trust in G-d and His creation.*

**Buddhist/Other Faiths:**

*Buddhism teaches, among other things, that solutions to problems and obstacles lie within our own bodies and minds- ourselves- not outside of our selves.*

*We believe a disease is a problem or an obstacle that must be resolved or overcome. The solution to this problem is a cure, or a successful resolution, to the disease, condition or physical crisis. The cure lies within our own bodies, our judgment or our family, The solution is not a vaccination from an outside source. Vaccination lies outside of the self. Clearly and absolutely, vaccines do not fit with the Buddhist religion and our personal translation of it.*

*The Buddhist faith also teaches purity of the mind in order to eliminate, hate, greed and ignorance. We believe the purity of the mind cannot be achieved without purity of the body and for this reason we forgo vaccines. We recognize, through the interpretation of our Buddhism beliefs, that vaccines make the body impure.*

**You may/may not want to explain why vaccines are different than other medical interventions that might be needed in a crisis for sick people.**

*I see a clear difference between helping a body in crisis and addressing a healthy body with medical help or intervention. (Refer to past explanations) Generally speaking, if my body were in crisis, I would consider all the options and discuss what to do with my trusted physician/healer. I would also consult with the Bible, pray to their God for help and guidance, consult with clergy and rely on the healing power of God to aid me..*

*Whatever God sends my way, I will seek His help for solutions and guidance. And my decisions will adhere to my personal belief in God.*

*I do not turn my back on all 'modern' medicine and its practices and philosophies. There is a significant difference between a body in crisis needing help and a body that is healthy accepting a medical procedure. I believe God would accept the former, He would not accept the latter.*

**You may/may not want to address the societal/institutional pressure to vaccinate as conflicting with your beliefs in the Higher Law of God:**

*The medical establishment as well as most friends and family apply pressure and guilt to others in society to participate in the vaccination process. Modern society tells us that we can hurt ourselves and other people if we do not accept this vaccine into our bodies. Society tells us we jeopardize babies, old people and everyone in between, if we do not vaccinate. Without a medical background or specific scientific knowledge, it is difficult to comment on the truth to that assertion. But the point is moot because I am certain of this; God has communicated to me that to address my flawless, healthy, God-given body with the procedure of vaccination would be a sin against my conscience.*

*The vaccination process has always created a feeling of anxiety and discord for me. However, I buried these feelings deep inside of me because there is so much pressure in society to vaccinate from family, friends and medical professionals. I let all this pressure hide the instinctual feeling I had that vaccination was simply contradictory to my bond with God.*

**End with the Emphasis on your *Personal Interpretation* Component and Reassert your Request for the Religious Exemption.**

You need to affirm the fact that the law allows you to have a personal religious belief that prohibits vaccination. This is the most important aspect of the law that enables virtually endless beliefs to fit squarely with the law.

*The above is an explanation of my sincerely held personal religious beliefs. I hope I have described them sufficiently. Again, these thoughts are the unique message I receive from my God. I don't ask that you, or anyone else, agree with these thoughts and personal translations.*
*But under the law, I respectfully request that they be honored as truthful and legally permissible.*
*Based on what I have shared, I ask this religious exemption be approved.*

EXAMPLE:

**Religious Vaccine Exemption Request**

[Your Name]

[Your Address]

[City, State, ZIP Code]

[Your Email]

[Your Phone Number]

[Date]

To Whom It May Concern,

I am writing to formally request a religious exemption from the vaccination requirements at [Name of School] for my child, [Child's Name]. As a practicing Christian with deeply held religious beliefs, I cannot, in good conscience, comply with this requirement. My faith compels me to uphold the sanctity of my body as created by God, and I firmly believe that vaccines violate these principles.

The Bible instructs us to honor and protect our bodies as temples of the Holy Spirit:

1 Corinthians 6:19-20 - "Do you not know that your body is a temple of the Holy Spirit within you, whom you have from God? You are not your own, for you were bought with a price. So glorify God in your body."

Furthermore, Scripture warns against the use of substances that may defile or alter the body that God has designed:

Leviticus 17:11 - "For the life of the flesh is in the blood, and I have given it for you on the altar to make atonement for your souls, for it is the blood that makes atonement by the life."

Psalm 139:13-14 - "For you formed my inward parts; you knitted me together in my mother's womb. I praise you, for I am fearfully and wonderfully made. Wonderful are your works; my soul knows it very well."

As followers of Christ, we are also called to trust in God for our health and well-being, rather than relying on human interventions that may conflict with our beliefs:

Jeremiah 17:7 - "Blessed is the man who trusts in the Lord, whose trust is the Lord."

Additionally, my conscience and faith reject any medical intervention that is connected to abortion-derived cell lines, as the Bible clearly states:

Exodus 20:13 - "You shall not murder."

Ephesians 5:11 - "Take no part in the unfruitful works of darkness, but instead expose them."

It is my firm conviction that participating in a vaccination program, particularly one that involves any connection to fetal cell research or potential harm to my God-given immune system, violates my religious
beliefs.

My faith commands me to act according to my conscience, and I respectfully request that this exemption be granted in accordance with my constitutional rights and religious freedoms.

I appreciate your time and consideration in reviewing my request. Please feel free to reach out if further discussion is needed.

Sincerely,

[Your Name]

I think it's important to realize that if we think refusing vaccinations is difficult now, it is only going to become more difficult in the future if we do not stand up against those trying to enforce the agenda.

# WHAT'S COMING

The Plan (Agenda) to Vaccinate the whole world:
https://www.hhs.gov/sites/default/files/vaccines-federal-implementation-plan-2021-2025.pdf

Cell Tower Radiation IS a Thing, and it's NOT Going Away Any Time Soon.
https://childrenshealthdefense.org/defender/telecom-industry-not-required-accommodate-people-sickened-cell-tower-radiation-courts-rule/

https://childrenshealthdefense.org/defender/marcia-haller-cell-tower-rf-radiation-sickness/

How Much Damage is Being Produces by Vaccines?
https://www.midwesterndoctor.com/p/how-much-damage-has-mass-vaccination

The Continual Attempt at Silencing, protecting the Narrative and Exploiting the Public
https://www.midwesterndoctor.com/p/the-price-of-truth-vs-deception-in?utm_source=publication-search

~

Matthew 24:30-39, 42-51, John 5:20-30, 1 John 2, Revelation

# More Stories:

## MMR ETC.

The day my son received the MMR vaccine, our lives changed forever. As we were walking out of the doctor's office, he suddenly froze in my arms, his body stiff, unresponsive, stuck to my shirt. I had to peel him off of me. In that moment, I thought my child had died.

Panic set in. They rushed him away from me while I was pulled into another room and questioned—as if I had done something wrong, while he lay there in recovery from appeared to be a seizure.

Later, we were sent home. I opened his wellness book and saw a febrile seizure was quietly noted in his records—a complete lie. That wasn't a "fever seizure." That was a full-body shutdown, happening just moments after the shot. When I questioned it, we were fired from the practice.

Best thing that ever happened to us. If we had stayed in that broken system, we never would have found the answers nature already had waiting for us.

We Were Never Given Informed Consent

We weren't warned. We weren't given informed consent. It was just what you did "to protect the herd." It wasn't something you questioned. You trusted the doctors. You followed the schedule. You assumed it was safe.

No one told me my son could experience seizures, brain swelling, or anaphylaxis. But he would.

Yes, anaphylaxis. A life-threatening allergic reaction that would become part of our everyday reality. Deadly food allergies. Autoimmune disease. Constant battles with his health. A life of reversing what never should have happened in the first place.

The Truth About Measles, MMR, and Vaccine Risk

For all the fear-mongering about measles, here's what they don't tell you: In the last 25 years, there have been only 3 measles-related deaths. In that same time, the MMR vaccine has been linked to 166 deaths and 77,221 recorded adverse reactions. These aren't mild side effects—these are serious injuries like seizures, paralysis, brain swelling, anaphylaxis, and even measles itself, all listed in the vaccine insert. Read that again if you have buts....

And here's the kicker: Only 1-10% of vaccine injuries ever get reported. That means the real number of MMR-related deaths could be as high as 16,600.

And for all that risk, you're not even guaranteed protection. During the Disneyland measles outbreak, 31% of cases were in vaccinated individuals. The media loves to lump the "unknown" vaccination status in with the unvaccinated, but if you flip it and assume some of those people were actually vaccinated, the real number could be as high as 70%.

So, save your "vaccines save lives" stories for someone who hasn't had to watch their child struggle with 22 years of chronic health issues, life-threatening allergies, and autoimmune disease.

If you're wondering why our health is so messed up, start thinking for yourself. Ask questions. Stop being blindly led by a system controlled by the pharmaceutical industry. Because once you see the truth, you can't unsee it.

* Dated pic of me and my son at the Capitol in Hartford, trying to keep our religious rights to say no , because when you really dive into what they put in these injections, you will find God again. If you don't, reassess yourself.

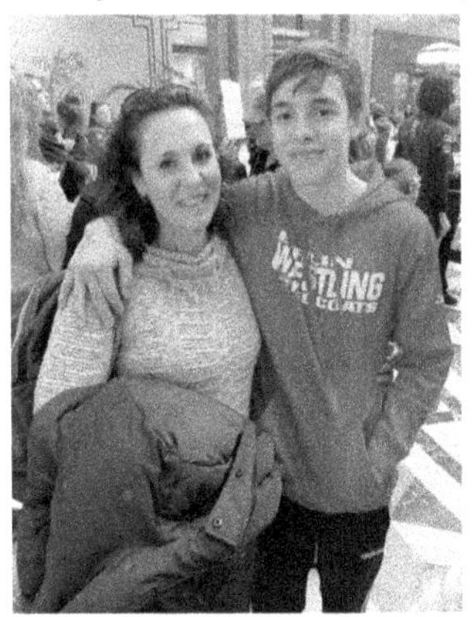

#mamabearhealthacademy
#masterkristenyousef
#WellnessWarriors
#noexcusesjustresults

Otto's Story

Joshua Coleman's son, Otto, was born perfectly healthy and developed normally. He met all milestones, had begun walking, climbing and even running. At around 15/16 months old, he had a well-baby visit on May 25th, 2010, and got 4 vaccine injections: Dtap, hib, prevnar13, and polio.

Soon after the shots, he started walking a little wobbly, but his parents thought he was just figuring his body out and still learning how to walk or just being silly. There was no real indication anything was wrong. Little did his parents know but Otto was losing muscle control.

And then one morning in early July, Otto woke up and couldn't move his legs, or walk at all.

They rushed him to the ER, where doctors ordered an MRI and spinal tap, and doctors diagnosed Otto with **transverse myelitis,** a neurological disorder caused by inflammation of the spinal cord.

Doctors brought up that this could be caused by either an airborne virus or vaccination. The Coleman family flew to Johns Hopkins Hospital where physicians there confirmed this to be a "one in a million" reaction to vaccines. Doctors told the family it was very rare, and the Coleman family believed it. Joshua did not start researching vaccines yet.

The Coleman's welcomed their second baby, and they gave him his first round of vaccines, but he got very sick. That's when the bells went off, and he started researching vaccines. He thought.... maybe there was something in their family's genetics that make them more susceptible to vaccine related injuries. Finally, he fell down the proverbial rabbit hole. And like any parent, he wanted to protect his children from being harmed again or treated differently for being susceptible to vaccine injury–which I think any parent would do if they found themselves in his circumstance.

Years later, Otto, now 12, is a typical pre-teen in every respect. He's into books and video games. While he did get minor sensation back in his legs, he did not get any muscle control, and he is still in a wheel chair.

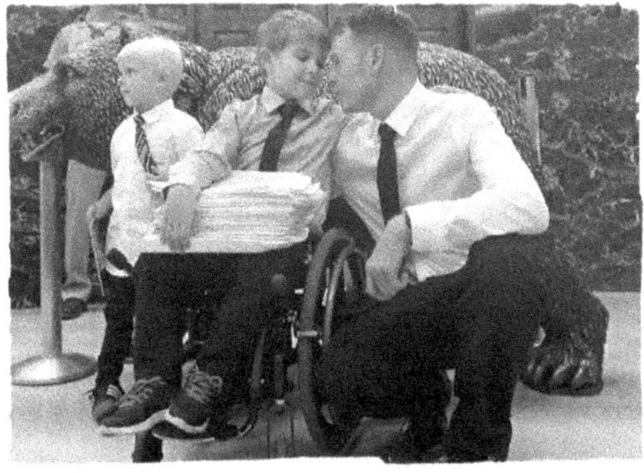

Hear Joshua Coleman's story in his own words:

https://circleofmamas.com/health-news/anti-vaccine-activist-spotlight-the-story-behind-the-signs-guy-joshua-coleman/

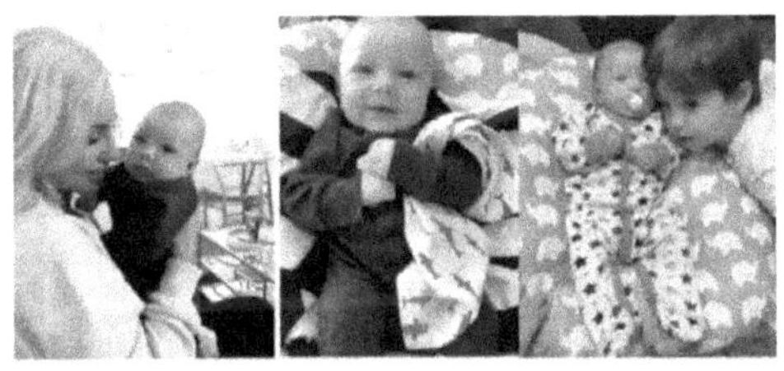

Brooks David Griffin

2/6/2021 - 5/20/2021

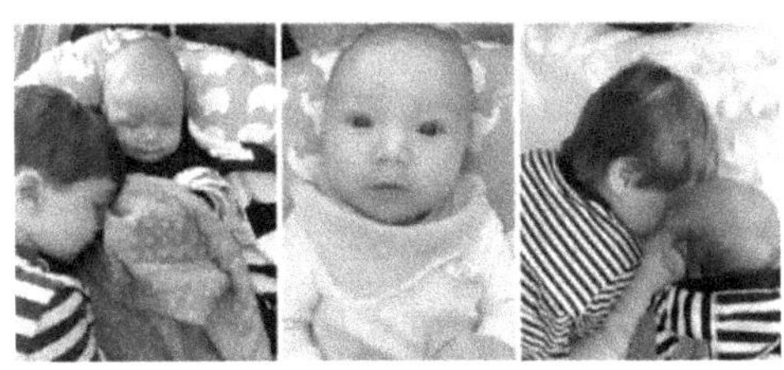

https://circleofmamas.com/health-news/baby-brooks-dies-suddenly-20-days-after-dtap-and-rotavirus-vaccines/

The Story of Kari Bundy's little boy, Mason's unnecessary death from vaccines after he was already sick. Please listen to this mother's cry to other mothers who are listening to their doctor's lethal advice. Watch Video Here.

https://www.facebook.com/watch?v=1168692554636174

## Mom Struggles with baby's Severe Skin Issues

Becoming a mom 4 years ago changed so many things for me but not how I felt health should be handled. I trusted my child's doctors and listened to their suggestions. We followed all the rules. Did everything "right." Took all advice. We got every vaccination. We ended up struggling with our first sons skin badly. Tried EVERY over the counter eczema treatment, creams, lotions, ointments. Tried all the steroids the doctors prescribed. Over and over. Higher and higher doses. Saw different specialists. With only very slight change to his skin. Our doctors suggested he would outgrow his skin issues and there was nothing to worry about, to just give it time...He went through complete steroid withdrawal. All the symptoms he previously had, he had worse, for several weeks. Finally recovering to his original state but not anywhere close to clear or comfortable.

At this point we became pregnant with our second son and after his birth we began to try and manage two children with skin conditions. After our second boys 2 month check up it was clear his was worse than our first. We decided NO steroids this time. We could not watch a second child go through such a terrible thing. By his 4 month check up we knew something was very wrong. But after several extra trips to the office, no one in the office agreed. So we switched doctors.

By this time he's having his 6 month appointment and got 7 vaccinations. Everything. Blew. Up. My precious baby was COVERED head to toe in rashes, pimples, scabbing. You name it, he had it. He couldn't sleep more than 30-45 minutes at a time because of how uncomfortable he was. Ripping the skin and flesh from his body and only stopping once you pulled his hands off of himself. This is not exaggerated, that was our real life for over a year. We saw allergists, dermatologists, dietitians, and multiple different doctors. As soon as we said we had a bad experience with steroids with our oldest and we wouldn't be using them again, we were immediately written off. After several more months of driving him all over the state seeing different medical professionals, getting testing done, popping positive for more than a dozen different allergens, several different rounds of antibiotics, trying new diets; dairy free, grain free, sugar free, they only gave us two answers, a $4,000/month out of pocket injection or steroids.

We felt so hopeless. Despite all our energy and resources being poured into our child's healing, he was absolutely miserable. His primary care doctor's response to this? Get him his next round of shots and hopefully he will grow out of it. Over a year of worsening symptoms and two offices she says sorry, hopefully he'll be fine If you didn't guess already, he got extremely worse. I was so angry and heartbroken. We never returned to the second office after that day and I decided to switch gears on a whim. I booked with a naturopath. I cannot stress enough how this SAVED MY SONS LIFE. Immediately looking at him she knew he needed to detox from heavy metals. (Something he had been tested for in the world of western medicine and I was assured he was fine). Yet he had high levels of several different kinds. We started detox. After everything we had went through, I'll admit I was skeptical. I had given up hope that it could be such an easy fix, but imagine that, he thrived. Almost instantly. He started being able to sleep, and without hand covers, then wear two piece outfits for the first time. He played in the dirt and swam in the lake, he grew drastically. Most importantly he was HAPPY!! For the first time in his short time here, he just got to be a kid.

Now? He's on a regular diet, eating all the foods he loves and growing by the second. None of the "allergens" are affecting him. We use NO over the counter creams/lotions. He sleeps ALL night long. Wrestles with his older brother. Most importantly, his skin is baby smooth for the first time in his life.♥ detoxing healed our entire family, I could not be more thankful every day I trusted myself more than the doctors.

I know the whole world is politically charged right now and there are some truly awful people making truly awful decisions for the rest of us but PLEASE remember my son. Injury and complication are REAL and much more COMMON than you think. Doctors are paid to care about you. My kids will probably never be able to attend public school because of this. I will be faced with the decision of their health or education because of this. Proceed with caution. I'm begging you.

*edit to add, many people have talked about the school waivers. I've been made aware that isn't the case everywhere but it is still very sad for the parents who are faced with that choice*

**edit: people asking what detox we used, this is not a one size fits all case and you need to seek help from a professional near you to best fit the needs of your child. We see Heather Dexter, if you're in the Grand Rapids area I cannot recommend her enough.**

Pictures from before and after. See for yourself. If you read this far, thank you.

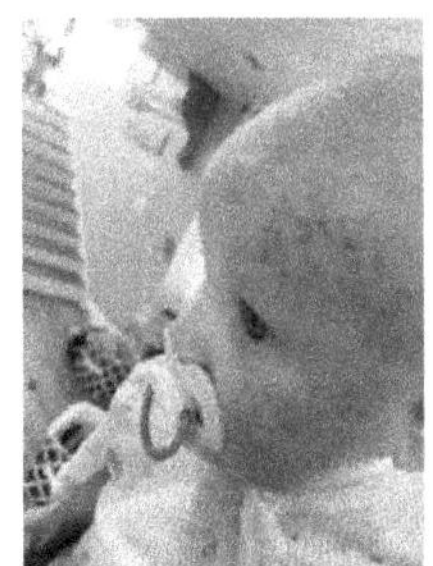 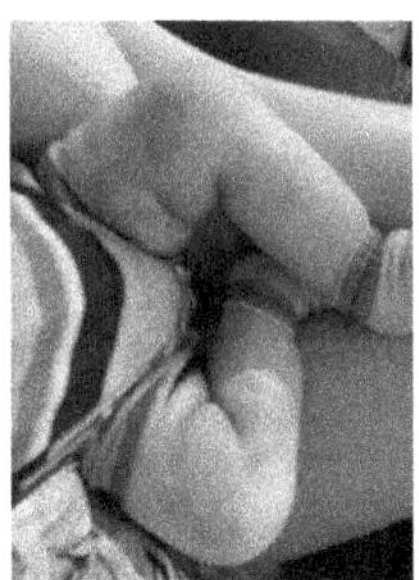 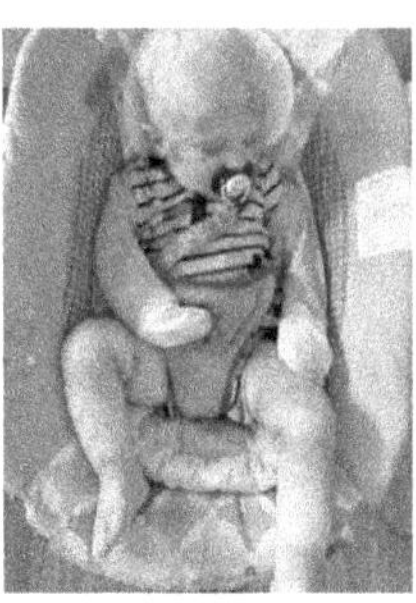 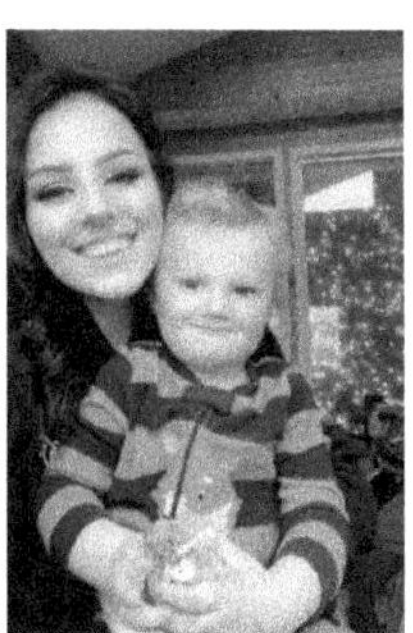

"Lauren Sikora is 31 years old .She has: Cerebral palsy

Epilepsy & Autism from a vaccine injury to her brain .

She was born normal.

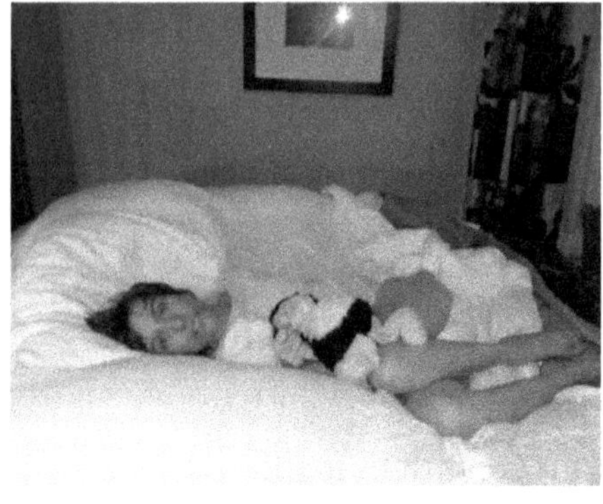

She cannot walk, talk or feed herself. Never could.

She got a DTP shot at 4 months old, then had a 15 minute long Grand Mal seizure afterwards; afterwards she was never the same.

Thimerosal crippled my sister.

Aluminum Hydroxide crippled my sister.

MSG crippled my sister. Formaldehyde crippled my sister.

Polysorbate 80 crippled my sister.

These are all in vaccines. DO NOT VACCINATE !

We are Lauren's Voice. She's my sister."

posted by Lauren's brother Joseph Sikora

Listen to this Nurse's story who learned the hard way to "listen to your inner mom voice", do the research and do not cave to the medical pressure.

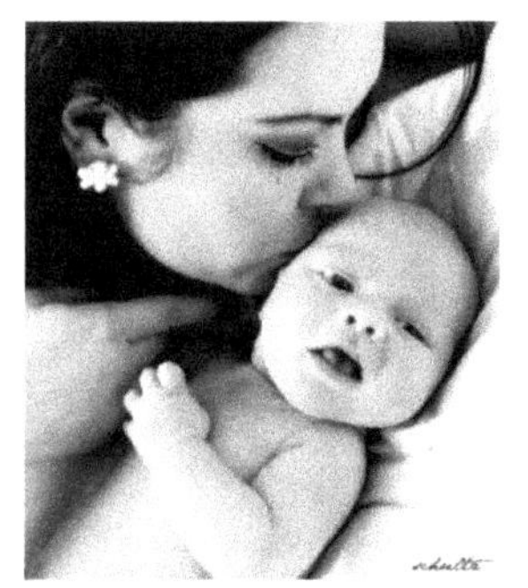

Monday Featured Spotlight: Angela Renee, BSN, RN

"It's been too long I have stayed silent. It's time to share my story. To speak the truth in love. My adult career as a Registered Nurse has been centered on the NICU, PICU, & Pediatric populations.

Growing up I had all my vaccines, the 11 or so we got back in 1984, seemingly unaffected and happily moving forward in life.

Fast forward to nursing school. I remember watching a short video, the CDC schedule & the importance of our patients receiving the full schedule. The denial of the autism link - and that's it. We did not study ingredients, we were not told about vaccine injury/death, or how to report to VAERS when an injury occurred. One class quickly spoon-fed. And we moved on.

Upon graduating and securing my first job in the NICU, I thought nothing of the injections I pushed into the thighs of my screaming newborn patients, nor of the "poor feeding," lethargy, high-pitched screams, & breathing abnormalities that would sometimes follow. This was all normalized as common for the short period after vaccines. I questioned nothing as my own belly grew and grew with my own first child. I was a nurse after all, and this was science.

I drove to my son's 2 months well visit and a voice inside told me, "Don't do it. You need to research first. " And I actually listened to my gut and declined. Me, the nurse who injected other people's babies...I told my pediatrician I just wanted to wait a bit and do some more research. I was made to sign a form acknowledging that I was putting my child at risk. I left feeling so shamed but relieved that there was still time to decide. Shortly after I received a phone call from my nurse manager that upon returning to work from my maternity leave, I would be joining the float pool which would place me returning to work in a brand new orientation to the pediatric and PICU units.

I returned to work reluctant to leave my newborn, also pregnant again with heavy morning sickness, and trying to learn a whole new patient population and 2 new units, with no time or leftover energy to do my vaccine research. And then the voices of my new nurse co-workers started sounding off: "You're crazy to not vaccinate your baby! You are working in a PEDS unit, don't you know how much risk you are putting him?!" They were well-intentioned, taught the same tiny tidbit as I was.

Well, I panicked. I dropped my resolve to research, left after work, and called my son's doctor. "I need an appointment as soon as possible for his vaccines because I work in pediatrics now, I can't put him at any further risk." And I went. And he screamed. Back at home, he was colicky, febrile, not feeding well, regurgitating large amounts of milk. I called the pediatrician's office. This was normal I was assured. It will pass. Duh, I knew that! And it did. I returned again for more shots at 6 months, 9 months, each time with similar reactions. Each time I brushed off that gut instinct that something was wrong, because, after all, the benefit of his protection outweighed the risk.

Time for the one-year vaccines, the plethora, the dreaded, accused MMR. This time with a newborn daughter in tow. But this time, was just too much. How I wish I could go back to that day I declined at 2 months and start my research then! How different things would be had I stood firm and learned back then what I know now. The toxic load of aluminum, formaldehyde, human and animal tissues, etc and etc, were too much for my son's neurological system and detoxification system. He lost his words & eye contact altogether, started flapping, spinning, walking on his toes, had horrible GI symptoms, food limiting, had no desire for social interaction, etc. He was diagnosed with severe autism. And our world was turned upside down.

I knew beyond a shadow of a doubt, before even starting my research, that the vaccines had triggered autism. I had watched it happen before my very eyes. No one could ever convince me otherwise. How sad to have to learn the hard way, when I was SO close to sparing my son a life of difficulty. Yet thankfully, unlike so many others, I still had HIM.

As I researched, I became more and more enlightened to the corruption, the cover-up, the lack of safety studies over 30 years, the politicians in league with the pharmaceutical companies, the secret tax-funded vaccine court with no liability of the manufacturers, following the money-trail as they say, and further down the rabbit hole, I went...Finding solace and comfort and support in those parents I met on this new journey who had also learned the hard way. Doctors, lawyers, teachers, educated professionals, now on a journey to try and recover their injured child, if they weren't mourning their loss, only to be met with scorn and mockery from those within their family and professional circle.

I went from fully supporting vaccines and administering them to others and my own children, to fully rejecting them and warning everyone who would listen, including my patients' parents, of the danger! I would even bribe my coworkers with snacks from the vending machine to administer vaccines to my patients that parents had signed for. I did not want any part in it, even if the parents wanted them given!

So my take-home message is, I get that you only want to protect your child, just as I did. I really do and I respect you for it! Us pro-vaxxers & Ex-vaxxers are NOT enemies! We all want the same thing - safety for our babies. So I don't want you to take my word for it. I hope that you'll heed my pain and do diligent research. It takes time. It is painful to uncover. But for every health professional reassuring, you vaccines are okay, you now have another rising up and telling you they are unavoidably, unequivocally UNSAFE. Please let that be the red flag to you, even if it is the ONLY red flag that causes you to dig deeper for yourself and your family.

Do you know why we are suddenly, and in such great numbers, stepping out of hiding, bearing the mockery, insults, wishes of death on us and our children?? (Yes, this is happening A LOT!)

It's because we can't afford to remain silent any longer, there is TOO much at stake for ALL of us!

~ 29 states currently are pushing legislation, that will ultimately remove ALLLL exemptions. Your right to choose for your children will first be taken. All 72 doses, including the HPV and flu vaccine mandated, with 270+ currently in the pipeline. Those will follow as soon as you no longer have any say so. Then they will come after us, the Adults.

Oh, you've been skirting around that monstrous flu vaccine each year? You won't be able to if you don't find the will to fight back now. You will be caught up on the same schedule our children are subjected to, and ALL the new ones as well. They just approved the HPV vaccine for adults! Make NO mistake, this IS the agenda. And it is happening rapidly.

So while we still have a chance, let's forget about pro-vax and anti-vax and stand together and fight for our right to CHOOSE ~ For autonomy over our own bodies and our children. Defend your CHOICE now, research later.

Where there is a risk, no matter how small, there MUST be a choice. Please stand and fight with us. We are being censored all over social media platforms and soon our voices will be silenced. We must awaken Now and stop allowing them to pit us against one another. For the sake of our children, grandchildren, our future. Get involved in your state, in any way you can, and fight with us for the right to keep your CHOICE. This is a civil liberties issue, NOT simply a vaccine issue. If we allow this, what's to stop them from force sterilizing or euthanizing, it's been done in the past! Then it will be forcing a chip that tracks everything. God bless you all and empower you with boldness. I am available in my inbox to lovingly answer questions."

♥ ~Angela Renee, BSN, RN

# Vaccine Damage Signs to look for.

**(from a fellow mom)**

**I can usually see the neurological damage on people's faces and it breaks my heart.**

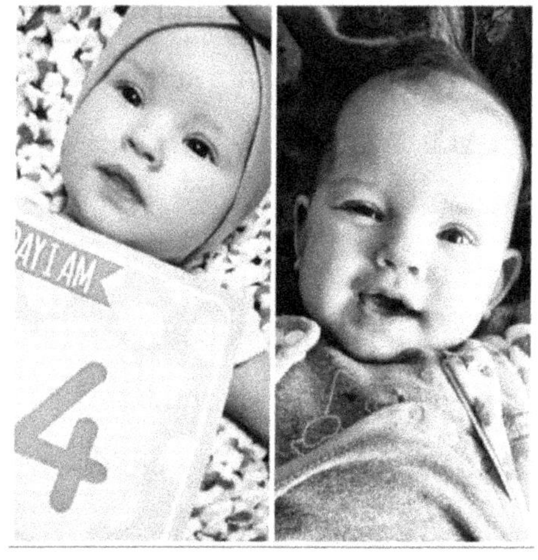


So far everyone I've seen who took the Covid shots or who are in close proximity to someone who did shows it. The book "Crooked: Man-Made Disease Explained: The Incredible Story of Metal, Microbes and Medicine — Hidden Within Our Faces" explains it well.

Evee's mom: "I've been hesitant to post this. Since Evee died, and the more research and cases I've read about, the more I've learned what was happening to my daughter in the 6 1/2 months of her life. This is not easy to acknowledge, much less accept. I'm only making this public to help another.

Evee was perfect. Beautiful. Smart. Funny. I now know that Evee had rather significant reactions to her shots that I didn't catch onto at all. After her Hep B and Vit K shot, her hematocrit increased. She had to be in and out of the lab for 2 weeks to keep track of it and make sure my breastfeeding helped to lower it in time, and it did.

2 month shots came along and after that, Evee started to do this head shaking, back and forth, back and forth, quickly. I thought it was to get herself to sleep, but it was after naps as well.

4 month shots came and the head shaking increased. She had the bad rash reaction on her hammies that everyone has seen. This is also when Evee's face became asymmetrical. Her right eye became "limp" permanently and she had a slant to her smile. 💔

I've researched the heck out of this. Dr. Andrew Moulden provided clear scientific evidence to prove that every dose of vaccine given to a child or an adult produces harm, neurologically. This sounds crazy, but shortly after this, he mysteriously died. True Story. 😔

Every reaction gets worse with the next vaxx given, Evee was injured from her first shot. I didn't see it because I had no idea. Evee had visible neurological damage to her face after 4 months. Evee shook her head constantly the day before she died. Her face was hot with those red cheeks, a rash they said it was. Her 6 month shots took her life, and that rash stayed with her after the rest of her body turned cold and pale. Even after her body was frozen before autopsy. 💔

This is what shots do. These are some things to look for. Remember, a rash one appointment, could mean you receiving a certificate of cremation after the next appointment. Please, parents, hear this well. 😢😱

Ugh that was a hard one to write."

**Link to Book: *Crooked: Man-Made Disease Explained: The incredible story of metal, microbes, and medicine - hidden within our faces.***

**By Forrest Maready**

https://a.co/d/8NMfLju

**Ongoing GARDASIL Damage**

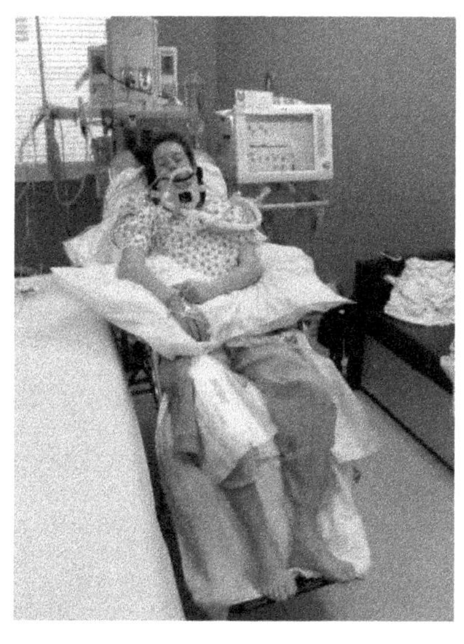

7 heartbreaking years ago my perfectly healthy son became a ventilator dependent quadriplegic due to the vaccine Gardasil.

Whether you call the condition TM or AFM they are both terms for polio renamed.

Colton fought so hard to get better. He was so strong and pushed himself trying to achieve a normal body that he once had, never to achieve it in this lifetime. Gardasil took his happy life from him. Gardasil took everything away from him that you take for granted like breathing, being able to walk, scratching your own itch, hugging someone, dressing yourself. Gardasil took my son from me. MERCK knows these risks exist. THE GOVERNMENT knows these risks exist Doctors know these risks exist yet they still administer vaccines because of money! They aren't administering vaccines for your health and safety it's all about money! There's no true safety studies on vaccines CDC destroys the info showing bad side effects from vaccines.

Please do your research...I did mine too late. My son is gone!

I miss him like crazy. You can protect your kids don't be a fool... don't trust a doctor that makes money pushing vaccines.

READ A TRUE VACCINE INSERT-DARE YOUR DOCTOR TO READ THE VACCINE INSERT. WHAT ARE THE INGREDIENTS= neurotoxins!

The HPV Vaccine On Trial: Seeking Justice for a Generation Betrayed (Colton's story is in this book! )

https://www.skyhorsepublishing.com/9781510710801/the-hpv-vaccine-on-trial/

Read this link to understand polio and how it's renamed!

https://truthbits.blog/2022/02/19/18-things-you-dont-know-about-polio/

His story is highlighted in *Vaxxed 2 the people's truth* on Peeps tv through Roku! [Link can be found on Children's Health Defense]

💔😭I miss you son💔😭💔

# CITED WORKS:

**[For Chapter 1 and some of 2]**

***Jenner and Vaccination: A Strange Chapter of Medical History***

By Charles Creighton M.D. London: Swan Sonnenschein & Co. Paternoster Square. 1889 Published by Andesite Press

This book is Public Domain

The same is also true of the next sighted work:

**[For Chapter 2]**

***The Evils of Vaccination, With a Protest Against its Legal Enforcement***

By George S. Gibbs

"Scholar Select" (22 pages) Printed in LaVergne, TN 12-10-23

**[For Chapters 3, 4, 5 and the "More Stories" sect. in Appx.]**

Most stories of personal injury are from shared FB posts and CircleofMammas.com website. (most stories along with their other sources are listed in the **Videos, Posts & FB LINKS sect**.)

**[For Chapter 4]**

DPT: Vaccine Roulette (1982) – (DPT: Diphtheria, Pertussis, and Tetanus Vaccines) Emmy Award winning documentary produced by Lea Thompson at WRC-TV in Washington DC in April 1982. (link in Vidoes, Posts & FB LINKS), **Vaccine Inserts** should be able to be found on the CDC's own website. The Inserts for the DTAP (Daptacel) and other Vaccines are from skool.com/pathtofreedom website in Classroom/ Medical Freedom section:

https://www.skool.com/pathtofreedom/classroom/ebc11a8f?md=8ac67b8f7f054e8680c2f12c47f7df25

**Studies of DPT in the 1980's**

https://www.sciencedirect.com/science/article/pii/S2352396417300464

MMR Insert Info:

https://www.skool.com/pathtofreedom/classroom/ebc11a8f?md=45ac395515ea4258808bef9d46f9c080

Dr. Toni Bark on Measles (Testifying in front of a House Committee Washington State.)

video clip on FB

https://www.facebook.com/search/top/?q=Dr.%20Toni%20Bark%20on%20Measles

Video on Rumble

Dr. Toni Bark's testimony at the Washington House Health Care & Welfare Committee Note: a few differences exist between the available, recorded speech and the [original transcript] some are noted by [brackets].

https://rumble.com/v2pzwke-dr.-toni-barks-testimony-at-the-washington-house-health-care-and-welfare-co.html?e9s=src_v1_s%2Csrc_v1_s_o

Study that showed that less than 1% of adverse events are ever reported to VAERS (or at least most likely)

https://rickjaffeesq.com/wp-content/uploads/2021/02/r18hs017045-lazarus-final-report-20116.pdf

G.A. Poland's Paradox of Measles

https://pubmed.ncbi.nlm.nih.gov/8053748/

**Recognizing Measles strains**

https://pubmed.ncbi.nlm.nih.gov/27852670/

Multitudes of studies sighted within the following article:

https://circleofmamas.com/measles/#MeaslesComplications

**Vit. K Insert Info:**

https://www.skool.com/pathtofreedom/classroom/ebc11a8f?md=5f5814402a1c418a91db677b6d1c5e6a

**Hep. B Insert Info:**

https://www.skool.com/pathtofreedom/classroom/ebc11a8f?md=15009f45904c4430bedf4c8cacf16a57

**On Polio:**

**Morton Biskind on DDT and the Real Cause of Polio**

https://www.westonaprice.org/health-topics/environmental-toxins/pesticides-and-polio-a-critique-of-scientific-literature/#gsc.tab=0

Original Article

https://canadahealthalliance.org/wp-content/uploads/2022/11/Pesticides-and-Polio_-A-Critique-of-Scientific-Literature-The-Weston-A.-Price-Foundation.pdf

**[For Chapter 5]**

https://www.news.com.au/sport/football/vaccine-theory-about-footballers-collapsing-debunked/news-story/013da222d688403b2568cc5e8404b1b0

**Story of Roy Butler who died shortly after COVID Jab:**

https://www.irishmirror.ie/sport/soccer/roy-butler-inquest-covid-vaccine-33743160?utm_source=mynewsassistant.com&utm_medium=referral&utm_campaign=embedded_search_item_desktop

**List of 69 Athletes dead after COVID Vaccine:**

https://dpbh.nv.gov/uploadedFiles/dpbhnvgov/content/Boards/BOH/Meetings/2021/Public%20Comments%20324%20to%20328.pdf

**The epidemiological relevance of the COVID-19-vaccinated population is increasing**

https://www.thelancet.com/journals/lanepe/article/PIIS2666-7762(21)00258-1/fulltext?s=08

***The Invisible Rainbow A History of Electricity and Life***

**By Arthur Firstenberg**

Published by Chelsea Green Publishing

White River Junction, Vermont, London, UK

Copyright 2017, 2020 by Arthur Firstenberg

Library of Congress Control Number: 2020930536

ISBN 978-1-64502-009-7

**Tamiflu Poisoning** Cited from: ***Virus Mania*** (p. 236-244)

***How the Medical Industry Continually Invents Epidemics, Making Billion-Dollar Profits at Our Expense***

By Torsten Engelbrecht; Cr. Claus Kohnlein, MD; Dr. Samantha Bailey, MD; Dr. Stephano Scoglio, BSc PhD 3rd Edition 2021

Published by Books on Demand

First published in 2007 by Trafford Publishing, All rights reserved

ISBN: 978-3-7526-2978-1

**Hep. C: *Virus Mania* (p. 169-178)**

**[For Chapter 6]**

Taken from Vaccine insert, general knowledge (cdc.gov, Mayoclinic.org etc.) and personal interpretation of observations.

**[Also Referenced in Chapters 5 and 6]** ***Virus Mania***

**[For Chapter 7]**

***Bechamp or Pasteur? A Lost Chapter in the History of Biology***

By Ethel D. Hume, First Published in 1923

***Pasteur: Plagiarist, Imposter The Germ Theory Exploded***

By R.B. Pearson, First Published in 1942

This edition copyright 2017 by: A Distant Mirror

ISBN-10 1467900125 ISBN-13 978-1467900126

**[For Chapter 8]**

Referenced: Plague by Judy Mikovits and Kent Heckenlively, Feb. 21, 2017 by Skyhorse Publishing ISBN-13 978-1510713949

Dell Bigtree's comments on measles Aired March 6th 2025

https://thehighwire.com/ark-videos/del-addresses-the-rfk-jr-measles-op-ed/

Description of Monoclonal Antibodies

https://pmc.ncbi.nlm.nih.gov/articles/PMC8521504/

New RSV Vaccine recommended

https://www.usatoday.com/story/news/health/2025/06/26/rfk-jr-acip-vote-rsv-shot-babies/84366939007/

Tucker Carlson's Interview with Dr. Patrick Soon-Shiong

https://www.youtube.com/watch?v=mgZaT-OriO8&t=2189s

**[For Chapter 9]**

Patient Counseling Information:

https://www.fda.gov/files/vaccines%2C%20blood%20%26%20biologics/published/package-insert-recombivax-hb.pdf

Chart of Vaccine Risk vs. Disease from the website of

https://vaccinechoicecanada.com/

Shared from Sarah Peterson's Skool/PathToFreedom website:

https://www.skool.com/pathtofreedom/classroom/ebc11a8f?md=429cc9899f20491f93971b28507f3382

Transcript of Dr. Lawrence Palevsky, (a Pediatrician practicing in Manhattan and on Long Island) discussing Connecticut's policies on required immunizations at a legislative informational Forum and the repeal of the religious exemption in NY, and the recent measles outbreaks. 11/22/2019

RFK on the MMR

https://healthimpactnews.com/2025/from-defending-childrens-health-to-destroying-it-robert-f-kennedy-jr-now-recommends-mmr-vaccine-after-years-of-condemning-it/

RFK fires 17 members of HHS

https://www.usatoday.com/story/news/health/2025/06/10/cdc-acip-members-terminated-rfk-vaccines/84134755007/

[For Chapters 5, 6, 8 & 10 (as well as throughout)]

Note: Much of these chapters are my own hypothesis, explanations and reasoning, as well as personal stories and observations on the matter.

## PICTURES

Picture of Charles Creighton

https://commons.wikimedia.org/wiki/File:Portrait_of_Charles_Creighton._Wellcome_M0010130.jpg

Picture of Physician Inoculating child

**https://commons.wikimedia.org/wiki/File:Doctor_vaccinating_a_young_child._Wellcome_M0002840.jpg**

Doctor vaccinating a young child after L. Boilly, 1827.

Wellcome Images

Picture of Edward Jenner: Edward Jenner, 1749-1823

*National Library of Medicine #101419674*

Picture of Protest Pic: No Vaccine Mandate

https://commons.wikimedia.org/wiki/File:Protester_at_protest_against_vax_mandate_protest_holding_sign_with_message_%22No_forced_vaccine%22_(51693638726).jpg

**Thalidomide effects.jpg**
https://commons.wikimedia.org/w/index.php?search=thalidomide+effects&title=Special%3AMediaSearch&type=image

Original Picture of Thalidomide children conglomeration:
https://www.instagram.com/p/CQrtuNGBbZ2/?utm_source=ig_web_copy_link

Much of the Info for Stories, other articles, information and opinions are from Facebook posts, and from

https://circleofmamas.com/

https://vaccineimpact.com/

https://steemit.com/

https://healthimpactnews.com/

https://vaccineresistancemovement.org/

https://aapsonline.org/

https://www.nvic.org/

https://childrenshealthdefense.org/

https://righttorefuse.org/

https://www.hhs.gov/sites/default/files/vaccines-federal-implementation-plan-2021-2025.pdf

https://worldpopulationreview.com/state-rankings/vaccine-exemptions-by-state#title

Appendices and More Information

For Drafting Religious Exemptions

https://ca.childrenshealthdefense.org/wp-content/uploads/Drafting-a-Religious-Exemption-Ltr-webfinal.pdf

Sarah Peterson's Inf on Vaccines from her Path to Freedom WP

https://www.skool.com/pathtofreedom/classroom/ebc11a8f?md=7242ab02a3f140a2b3fc9058b7caced0

Lawsuits for Gardasil/HPV vaccine injuries/deaths

https://www.thelibertybeacon.com/feds-sued-for-secrets-on-hpv-vaccine-deaths/

Aiden's Story with various studies sited:

https://circleofmamas.com/health-news/measles-rash-and-35-minute-seizure-9-days-after-vaccines-aidens-story/

Study on NIH National Library of Medicine

A 2021 Geier and Geier longitudinal study reported:

Childhood MMR Vaccination and Seizure Disorder

https://pubmed.ncbi.nlm.nih.gov/32981784/

Note: On fig. 1 Data for Unvaccinated children was from a Larger pool of children, and also reports of seizure disorder of those vaccinated with MMR were ONLY reported from days 6-11 after initial dose. It also failed to recognize any possible seizure related issues from other vaccines.

Article on Vaccine Schedule throughout history

https://circleofmamas.com/health-news/the-vaccine-schedule-through-the-years/

About Gardasil

https://circleofmamas.com/vaccine-inserts/

https://circleofmamas.com/hpv-human-papillomavirus/

# Other Books for Reference Tools and Further Research:

***The Contagion Myth*** By Cowen and Morell

***Dissolving Illusions***
***Disease, Vaccines, and the Forgotten History***
By Suzanne Humphries, MD and Roman Bystrianyk

## List of Books on the History of Vaccines for Further research:

1) The Poisoned Needle: Suppressed Facts About Vaccination Eleanor McBean, PhD, ND 1957
2) A Century of Vaccination and What It Teaches William Scott Tebb, MA, MD, DPH 1898
3) Vaccination: Proved Useless and Dangerous From 45 Years of Registration Statistics Alfred R. Wallace, LLD DUBL., DCL OXON., FRS, etc. 1885
4) Vaccination: Its Fallacies and Evils Robert A. Gunn, MD 1882
5) Compulsory Vaccination: The Crime Against the School Child Chas. M. (Charles Michael) Higgins 1915
6) The Truth about Vaccination and Immunization Lily Loat, secretary of the National Anti-Vaccination League of London 1951

7) Leicester: Sanitation versus Vaccination Its Vital Statistics Compared with Those of Other Towns, the Army, Navy, Japan, and England and Wales By J.T. Biggs, J.P. 1912

8) The Vaccination Question Arthur Wollaston Hutton, MA 1895

9) Vaccination a Delusion: Its Penal Enforcement a Crime Alfred Russel Wallace, LLD DUBL., DCL OXON., FRS, etc. 1898

10) Vaccination a Curse and Menace to Personal Liberty With Statistics Showing Its Dangers and Criminality James Martin Peebles, MD, MA, PhD Tenth Edition, 1913

11) Dr. C.G.G. Nittinger's Evils of Vaccination C. Charles Schieferdecker, MD 1856

12) The Vaccination Question in the Light of Modern Experience An Appeal for Reconsideration C. Killick Millard, M.D., D.Sc. 1914

13) Jenner and Vaccination: A Strange Chapter of Medical History Charles Creighton, MD 1889

14) The Horrors of Vaccination: Exposed and Illustrated Charles M. Higgins 1919

15) Vaccination: The Story of a Great Delusion William White 1885

16) Vital Statistics in the United States, 1940-1960 Robert D. Grove, Alice M. Hetzel US Department of Health, Education, and Welfare 1968

17) The Mandatory Vaccination Plan National Immunization Policy Council 1977

18) The Fraud of Vaccination Walter Hadwen, JP., MD, LRCP., MRCS, LSA From "Truth," January 3, 1923

19) Vaccination a Curse C.W. Amerige, MD 1895

20) Vaccination a Medical Fallacy Alexander Wilder, MD 1879

21) The Dream & Lie of Louis Pasteur Originally Pasteur: Plagiarist, Imposter R.B. Pearson 1942

22) The Vaccination Problem Joseph Swan 1936

23) The Fallacy of Vaccination John Pitcairn, President of the Anti-Vaccination League of America 1911

24) The Case Against Vaccination Walter Hadwen, JP, MD, LRCP, MRCS, LSA 1896

25) A Catalogue of Anti-Vaccination Literature The London Society for the Abolition of Compulsory Vaccination 114 Victoria Street, Westminster 1882, 2018

26) Never Vaccinate Your Child Lessons from Parents, Doctors, Scientists, Media, and HISTORY Trung Nguyen June 2018

# Videos, Posts & FB LINKS

The Triplets: Richie, Clair & Robbie, who get autism on the same day: FB Post by Nick Catone

https://www.facebook.com/watch/?v=603548869820112

Video Link:

https://steemit.com/vaxxed/@truthisterrorism/healthy-triplets-went-in-for-vaccine-shots-all-3-got-autism-that-day?fbclid=IwY2xjawI7B-pleHRuA2FlbQIxMAABHaWoaID3LOc3r5qUm4mITDjsd6_OBMmaC99ILoRjRshkJ7cctR5OG5mpdQ_aem_zfIaADBTfEgbW9m_Imqx5g

More FB Posts by Nick Catone

https://www.facebook.com/officialnickcatone/videos/1485724414807972

Story from Cilla Bugg: the nurse who was Willow's Mom

https://www.facebook.com/cillajilks/posts/pfbid02NLNcnX6MMRDrv3QNrj6ujxpqjovkc8PDEWDzQvf3TCsf385rhebvtE2Rh99Vhtu8l?__cft__[0]=AZXHfYF947cwioC61LYQs1Oj2gxtE5lMZqHaYq_qVo87duypfYhTRJs-ikKR1yCnc0LbLganPLw4WHN0-jvlMd6_LJMjbbSod6LjHVwjgysXsGIuFi8GyHuPpCty6KYqZx9EWpNA90GjRdgPe1lzE8lV72MFN5dAyt7PCyLQJ_XWAg&__tn__=-UK-R

Baby with Measles

https://www.facebook.com/photo?fbid=1496798927033854&set=a.1389054904474924

Story of Chris Runquist' twin daughters Jessica and Ashley

https://www.facebook.com/share/p/16ZodyuR18/

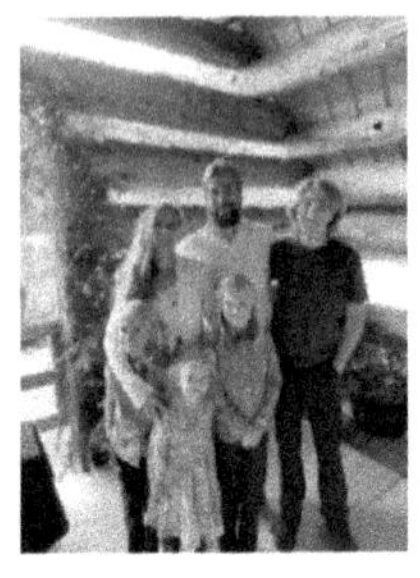

This is David's Facebook page:

https://www.facebook.com/david.stephan.568

## Videos

You can view The Story of The People Vs. David and Collet Stephen and watch the film at:

https://matadorfilms.ca/?fbclid=IwY2xjawI9ZeFleHRuA2FlbQIxMAABHVWWne8kOx334N--MnwoOBoHg47ObB-lDPQ1V2cYaHkeZGDpkE27tyCAHg_aem_aSIG0Vn2qHkKyqpNJcG11Q

Baby Nash

https://www.bitchute.com/video/VeCJhIZBXt7p

Shots In The Dark Silence on Vaccine - Full Documentary

https://www.bitchute.com/video/tLPWqVLzSVh4/?fbclid=IwY2xjawI55BtleHRuA2FlbQIxMAABHbmKm_iCfypAFQ1gnJHjBU3ix96pd6gnO7801xsNNgvlkNESkA3D6HRKaw_aem_7XosTbpksJkU9UfX6bOIRw

News Story of Nick Catone

https://newjersey.news12.com/former-professional-fighter-says-vaccines-are-to-blame-for-sons-death-38999281

Nick Catones's FB Site

https://www.facebook.com/officialnickcatone

DPT: Vaccine Roulette 1982

https://www.bitchute.com/video/REjyEwRk7qC3

Watch the Video presentation and view info related to the triplets who acquired autism all on the same day:

https://steemit.com/vaxxed/@truthisterrorism/healthy-triplets-went-in-for-vaccine-shots-all-3-got-autism-that-day?fbclid=IwY2xjawI0k7tleHRuA2FlbQIxMAABHXgb38hn2DrQuriTG3w7oSMwUVvbPZSbzIB11x6p-PfL34syOvjeEw9DSw_aem_EnbxaDznoTPB0YzZ2whmog

Post about How Vaccines Cause Autism

https://www.midwesterndoctor.com/p/how-do-vaccines-cause-autism?fbclid=IwY2xjawJJtVVleHRuA2FlbQIxMAABHYkmeKgjQ-R4c1x86Yrnui4Lg4X-rP_ZK90hotlBVxNt8QKel3B4GPpUOw_aem_PZw-gddVgrzKDgEOS5YbLA

## On the MMR

References for vaccine failures in vaccinated populations or measles outbreaks caused by vaccine strain in vaccinated populations:

https://www.science.org/content/article/measles-outbreak-traced-fully-vaccinated-patient-first-time

There is a great amount of information on measles from this sight: https://circleofmamas.com/measles/#MeaslesComplications

Note: much Info. is taken from medical journals such as The National Library of Medicine

MOG Disease and Vaccines

**Measles-rubella vaccine**-associated MOG-antibody positive acute demyelinating encephalomyelitis with optic neuritis in a child

Myelin oligodendrocyte glycoprotein antibody-associated disease following **DTaP vaccination**: A case report

MOG encephalomyelitis after **vaccination** against severe acute respiratory syndrome coronavirus type 2 (SARS-CoV-2): case report and comprehensive review of the literature

Myelin Oligodendrocyte Glycoprotein Antibody Disease After **COVID-19 Vaccination** – Causal or Incidental?

Unilateral optic neuritis after **vaccination** against the coronavirus disease: two case reports

ON GARDACIL and OTHER VACCINES

**http://vaccineresistancemovement.org**

**Watch an interview with Isabella's mother Kristine on Children's Health Defense.**

**Link pasted here:** Mothers of 2 Girls Who Died After Gardasil HPV Vaccine Sue Merck • Children's Health Defense

Or visit:

https://childrenshealthdefense.org/defender/gardasil-sydney-figueroa-isabella-zuggi-hpv-vaccine-lawsuits-deaths/

1) TLB recommends you visit: www.wnd.com for more great articles and information.

See original here: **http://www.wnd.com/2013/03/feds-sued-for-secrets-on-hpv-vaccine-deaths/#bVPPI4L758Z3teJS.99**

2) TLB recommends you visit: www.judicialwatch.org for more great articles and information.

See original here: **http://www.judicialwatch.org/press-room/press-releases/hpv-vaccine-injuries-and-deaths-is-the-government-compensating/**

Brianne Dressen's Story

Her Story on Fox News:

https://www.foxnews.com/politics/inhumane-utah-mom-slaps-drug-company-lawsuit-after-suffering-covid-vaccine-trial-injuries

With Shane Smith

https://www.bing.com/videos/riverview/relatedvideo?q=Brianne+Dressen&mid=465F5293A9A5A0F6BC38465F5293A9A5A0F6BC38&FORM=VIRE

Story on Rumble with Advertisement for her book about her story: *Worth a Shot*

https://rumble.com/v6qmqiy-i-was-injured-in-the-covid-vaccine-trials-and-still-struggle-every-day-bria.html

At Washington DC

https://www.youtube.com/watch?v=K3OdHFvu8jY&t=179s

The original link to Dr. Palevsky's speech
https://healthimpactnews.com/2020/dr-lawrence-palevsky-testimony-unvaccinated-children-are-thehealthiest-children-i-have-ever-seen/
(It has since been removed)

# VAXXED Documentaries:

## Taken from The Children's Health Defense website

VAXXED

https://live.childrenshealthdefense.org/chd-tv/videos/vaxxed-from-cover-up-to-catastrophe-movie/?fbclid=IwY2xjawJJsaZleHRuA2FlbQIxMAABHf1MFO725nDC_rejAaThaRsr5mouQFxCPaC7LRX3vn0PFgOYvSvF6icy4A_aem_yxu4Ns3Y3JtxjzCycNonOQ

VAXXED 2

https://live.childrenshealthdefense.org/chd-tv/videos/vaxxed-2/?fbclid=IwY2xjawJJsd5leHRuA2FlbQIxMAABHXRSatHV_Bd80c59zFCCmWvVcPk3wTR_R6kbKpuGuGUqUu4shss9xpzD4w_aem_GZCIIUdCtoOSjQDx5aAZYA

VAXXED 3

https://live.childrenshealthdefense.org/chd-tv/videos/vaxxed-3-or-authorized-to-kill-movie/?fbclid=IwY2xjawJJshlleHRuA2FlbQIxMAABHfyqp_i_SKuQbIcIakHVKr4kNJFO9HS8z54nuppJOiVoA1MBns2mYAAqrA_aem_ef4mrrmV6FzOPiNTindkmQ

Recent article from midwesterndoctor.com about

# VACCINE SHEDDING
# Unraveling the Mysteries of mRNA Vaccine Shedding

How is it possible and what can you do about it?

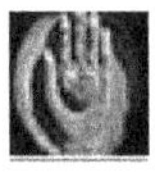

A Midwestern Doctor

Jan 21, 2024

**Story at a Glance:**

Over the last two years, we have collected a significant amount of data that suggests a sizable number of unvaccinated people will become ill around individuals who were vaccinated in a fairly consistent and repeatable manner.

Since shedding of mRNA vaccines in theory should not be possible, whenever those individuals (who are often suffering immensely) share their stories, they are immediately ridiculed and dismissed.

We have identified a few plausible mechanisms (and the evidence to support them) to explain why this transmission occurs. These include exosome mediated shedding (most likely), asymptomatic COVID-19 shedding and transfected bacterial shedding.

In this article, we will explore some of the greatest concerns surrounding shedding, such as what's currently known about sexual shedding, the odor some notice shedders emit, receiving vaccinated blood transfusions, cancer and shedding, and the existing methods which can be used to mitigate the harmful effects of shedding.

After the COVID vaccines came out, we began to encounter more and more patients who had a compelling case history that suggested that were being repeatedly injured from being around recently vaccinated individuals. For example, near the start of the vaccine rollout, a compelling (but hard to believe) story circulated online and as the year went by, we saw more and more patients who provided similar accounts to the one within this video:

Video shows the testimony of young girl who is extremely sensitive to those who have been vaccinated with mRNA vaccines, to the point of experiencing detox symptoms so badly she is afraid to go out in public.

I recommend viewing the three minute video for yourself.

(See link at the end of article)

All of this perplexed us as in theory, the mRNA vaccines (as they are not alive and hence do not replicate) should not be able to shed, but as time went forward, we kept on seeing more shedding cases which symptomatically improved once the patient's shedding exposures were addressed. As a result, we've spent the last three years struggling to try to figure out what's going on.

To help unravel this mystery, we recently put out a call for individuals to share their own shedding injuries and see if those accounts matched what we had observed. These is understandably a lot of interest in this subject (e.g., a Tweet about it received 555k views) and we've now collected hundreds of stories (which can be viewed here).

To briefly summarize what we have learned (which is discussed in much more detail in the previous article):

- Although it is required by the FDA (and has been done for the other gene therapy products on the market), none of the COVID vaccines were ever tested for shedding.
- It has since been demonstrated that vaccine sheds in the breast milk and semen. There is also evidence suggesting but not proving the vaccine sheds in both the sweat and breath. It's much less clear if it sheds in the stools.
- Individuals appear to be affected by being in proximity to a vaccinated person (particularly if they are quite close to them), by touching something a vaccinated person contacted (particularly bed sheets), and for particularly sensitive individuals, being in an area which had previously been densely occupied by shedders (conversely being outdoors, presumably due to airflow, reduces how much a shedder affects someone nearby).
- In most (but not all) cases, the effects of shedding will resolve once the affected individual simply stops being in contact with shedders.
- The susceptibility to shedding greatly varies person to person (with the majority not being affected by it). Those most sensitive to shedding are the "sensitive patients" (who often also have other conditions like fibromyalgia, Lyme or chemical sensitivities), those who have already been "sensitized" to the spike protein (demonstrated by them having either a vaccine injury or long COVID) and those who

have a yet unknown susceptibility to the spike protein (which I believe is due to them being unable to effectively produce antibodies which neutralize the spike protein). *Note: there were also a few cases of pets being affect by shedding which suggests the effects are not necessarily dependent upon a human receptor.*

- Individuals are the most likely to shed immediately after vaccination or boosting (which leads to many sensitive individuals dreading the next boosting campaign). This tendency to shed appears to match the observed blood levels of spike protein which quickly rise following vaccination then drop, but never hit zero. In turn, the most sensitive individuals always notice if someone was vaccinated, while less sensitive individuals only get ill from people who had been recently vaccinated.
- Many individuals affected by shedding are able to identify clear reproducible patterns of when they get ill from shedding (e.g., each time they go to church on Sunday they get the same illness on Monday).
- Some people shed much more than others (e.g., individuals can frequently identify who at their church always makes them ill). Typically, younger people shed more than older people. Furthermore, sensitive individuals repeatedly notice certain characteristics of shedders (e.g., they have a distinct odor).
- The most common effect of shedding is abnormal menstrual bleeding (which can sometimes be very severe and

frequently affects post menopausal women). Other common symptoms include nosebleeds, spontaneous bruising, tinnitus, rashes, headaches, reactivation of latent viruses (e.g., shingles), briefly coming down with a covid like illness, sinus issues and muscle pain. Some people experience a cluster of these symptoms while others only experience one or two of them.

- Individuals tend to notice an increasing duration of exposure to a shedder will make them feel worse. In turn, numerous readers have noticed that if they ignore their lighter symptoms (which often onset within minutes of a shedding exposure) and do not exit the situation, they will become severely ill for a prolonged period.
- Most of the shedding injuries appear to be a consequence of circulatory impairments (e.g., microclotting). I personally believe this is due their adverse effects on the physiologic zeta potential (which once treated appears to fix spike protein injuries) and to a lesser extent activating the cell danger response.
- Most of the vaccine shedding symptoms resemble what is seen in other spike protein injuries. However, there are two key differences. First, spontaneous bruising and nosebleeds are unique to shedding (they are not typically seen after long COVID or a vaccine injury). Secondly, the symptoms which emerge from shedding exposures tend to be less severe than the traditional spike protein injuries (e.g., heart issues or strokes are rarer and less severe) and when the severe

effects occur (e.g., death), they are typically proceeded by less severe reactions to shedding (but unfortunately the victim continued to expose themselves to shedders).

This suggests that the shedding reactions are being caused by reactions to a lower dose of spike protein—which is congruent with the fact a vaccinated individual will have more spike protein inside them than what is shed into their environment.

- Shedding effects are typically either immediate (e.g., nosebleeds, headaches and dizziness), onset in 6-24 hours (e.g., menstrual issues) or gradually show up over time. *Note: none of these are absolutes (e.g., sometimes the nosebleeds take a day to manifest, whereas I found one case where someone had severe menstrual bleeding immediately after a shedding exposure).*
- Two studies have validated the shedding effect is real.
- The majority of people do not appear to be affected by shedding.

**Mysteries of the Shedding Phenomenon**

The previous facts understandably raise a lot of uncomfortable questions many want answers to (hence why we received so many replies). I personally believe they necessitate a federal law being passed which will prohibit any gene therapies from entering the market unless their shedding is properly evaluated, that data is made public and it can be proven it is feasible to prevent the general public from being shed on.

Given the gravity of this situation, we believe it critical to provide the most accurate and balanced assessment of the COVID vaccine "shedding" phenomenon. This in turn was why we put out a public call for as much information on it as possible and why we've been as transparent as possible in how we reached our conclusions and provided all the data we used that helped us reach this conclusion. Since mRNA "shedding" is such an inexplicable phenomenon, attempts to explain or predict it inevitably result in a large number of highly speculative hypotheses being raised. In turn, it was my hope that consistent patterns would be seen in the shedding reports which could narrow down which of those hypotheses could fit the observed patterns and hence were more likely to answer many of the questions which have been repeatedly raised on this subject. For the rest of the article as we attempt to untangle this mystery, I will share our current perspectives on what ***might*** be going on and the answers to the most commonly received questions on it.

**The Vaccine Smell**

One of the most surprising things I learned from exploring the shedding issue is how many people have reported observing a distinct smell from individuals who appear to shed [e.g., 1, 2, 3, 4, 5, 6, 7, 8, 9, 10, 11, 12, 13, 14, 15, 16, 17, 18, 19, 20, 21, 22, 23, 24, 25, 26, 27, 28, 29, 30, 31, 32]. Additionally, many also notice this smell is present in areas where many vaccinated individuals have been (e.g., after a booster rollout, in crowded public spaces, or inside cars they drove).

Overall, it appears that a higher spike protein load appears to be "easier" to smell (e.g., in someone recently vaccinated—as spike protein levels spike in the blood after vaccination, when in close proximity to a shedder particularly if some type of intimate contact occurred, or when around someone who for some reason has a greater degree of shedding). Similarly, more sensitive people (who are typically more likely to be injured by the vaccines) are more likely to detect this smell (e.g., they can still smell it once the shedders are are no longer physically present).

*Note: numerous readers reported being able to consistently tell if someone was recently vaccinated.*

Additionally, I've found a few cases where:

Secondary shedding could be smelled.

A sexual partner lost their distinctive odor.

At least one individual with a vaccine injury could smell the shedding on themselves. [e.g., 1, 2, 3]. I would like to quote what one of those individuals shared since I believe it may offer some vital clues for unravelling this mystery:

The smell was one of the first symptoms of my vax injury (albeit a benign one, compared to what it eventually turned into). It was like my entire smell changed. I was living in Florida at the time - needless to say I'd sweat a lot. And every time, post-vax, my underarm sweat would have this strange metallic smell.

I would complain to my girlfriend about it. Always telling her "there's just something off. I can sense it"... at the time, she wasn't picking up on it. Or she disagreed as to the nature of the smell, while begrudgingly agreeing there was a slight change (she thought I was overreacting; also, she is unvaccinated)....But then a friend pointed it out at a workout class when I was sweating heavily.

I've been on a number of therapies for over a year now. The smell comes and goes. When it comes, I know I'm in for a flare up. It seems the flare ups tend to come from shedding (both viral and synthetic shedding). I haven't noticed the smell on others. Just myself. It makes me feel like I'm not me anymore, and that I've been hijacked.

The labels I've seen used to describe the smell are as follows: "**mild sickly sweet**," "**rotting [or dying] flesh**," "magnetic onion," "unpleasant," "distinctive," "the smell of death," "medicines plus latrines" "**musty plus rancid**" "dead animal," a "decomposing body," "**road kill**," "like ammonia but not as strong," "**sweet**," "sour stomach" "elderly person as their flesh breaks down with age," "a chemical flu smell" "of seaweed," "putrid," "sweet meat" "**strange and metallic**" "sharp, pungent and toxic" "horrible" "unique odor" "**chemical**," "vinegar," "subtle like a pheromone."

*Note: bolded items were reported by multiple people.*

From looking at this list of smells, a few things jump out at me:

•While it's quite difficult to put into words something which has never been described before, the descriptions are fairly consistent with each other.

•One of the most well recognized consequences of the vaccination is accelerated aging, which appears to be reflected in this list.

**There may be two separate things people are smelling** (the decomposing flesh vs. the metallic chemical). One theory which was proposed to me to explain the second smell is that its a result of micro-organisms in the environment that have been metabolizing all the chemicals that were used to (pointlessly) sterilize every surface through COVID-19 as one reader said it was first noticed in 2020 but dramatically increased in 2021.

Individuals who can smell this will likely lose their attraction to shedders (as appealing smells are often the most important thing for sexual compatibility).

*Note: one sensitive person who can perceive the shedding has shared that they've completely lost their attraction to vaccinated women for this reason.*

The one friend I have who can smell this (and a very perceptive colleague) reports that it appears to be being emitted through the pores. This is consistent with what some of the individuals (e.g., the one quote above) observed and the evidence ***suggesting*** the shedding occurs through the sweat since it contaminates sheets.

Since individuals often perceive the same environmental quality through different senses (depending on their primary sensory orientation is) I was also curious to see other ways the "quality" shedders had was described.

Since smell is intimately linked to taste, I expected those reports to resemble the smells. The three I received [1, 2, 3] did just that, describing it as: "you can taste the jabs…it's metallic and unpleasant" "can taste a metallic sensation" "a dry acid feeling on my tongue."

Quite a few people also reported feeling sensations from vaccinated individual [e.g., 1, 2, 3, 4, 5, 6, 7, 8, 9] and described them as follows: "noxious," "recently vaccinated people have a slime on their skin" "it was a feeling of repellent that made me want to get away as quickly as possible," "the bioelectric field around the person disappears," "their energy changes to a stainless steel sink sponge feel which is metallic and raggedy (which that reader ***believed*** represented neurologic damage)" "illness and excitable energy" "a heavy air pressure and spatial fog weighing on my brain (which if not exited from will then create vertigo for that reader)," "it makes our noses prickle," "half of my tongue went numb the next day" "their energy field has a physical sensation of 'metallic' of physical repulsion, or a greyness, black goo, and even a dullness of mind that I could see"

*Note: the last commenter also noted they verified they could accurately predict who was vaccinated and that they noticed food prepared from vaccinated individuals was different.*

As you might notice, these are somewhat congruent with the previously described smells and tastes.

One sensitive physician I know who smells the odor (and seems to know more about it than anyone else I know) has shared the following with me:

•They had previously had environmental sensitivities, which with work they were able to eliminate.

•Until those sensitivities were resolved, they would smell chemical residues on them when they got home which they then needed to clean off.

•In December 2020 (right after the rollouts began), they began to notice a new smell they'd never smelled before which lingered on them once they got home and they needed to clean off (e.g., with a shower) in order to be able to be comfortable at home (previously, while sensitive, they'd also needed to do this for everyday chemical exposures).

•Before long, this smell started emerging in public places (e.g., a store), but was by far the strongest in the hospital. Because this smell had not existed throughout the first year of the pandemic, they assumed it was linked to the vaccine. Presently, they believe the smell is the spike protein and something else in the vaccine.

•The smell gets stronger each time a new series of boosters is rolled out (as most of coworkers at the hospital likely receive it).

•This smell was much weaker in Southern Europe, suggesting either their vaccines were different, or the health of the average American caused them to shed differently.

•When the shedding smell is particularly strong, they experience temporary symptoms while around those individuals (e.g., pain in a part of the body). This for instance occurred after the most recent round of boosters.

•Many people who were vaccinated do not have this smell, which suggests many (as discussed in the previous article) received placebos. Unfortunately for my colleague, it is much higher in hospitalized patients (which suggests those who received the more potent vaccines were also more likely to be injured and hence hospitalized). Likewise, the more "real" doses someone received, the harder it is for my colleague to be around them.

*Note: presently my colleague estimates around 50% of the population is truly jabbed, but in certain cases (e.g., in clinics for the elderly who are more likely to have been repeatedly boosted, this figure rises to 80%). Sadly, those with the most unusual or severe illnesses, they invariably muscle test (or smell) as having been "truly" vaccinated. The subject of "hot lots" has been a longstanding controversy*

•The mold biotoxin community has also noticed a new toxin (and odor) they need to be wary of which entered the environment during 2020 and worsened in 2021 after the vaccines hit the market. Likewise, my colleague has had patients who believed they'd had a mold exposure (which is often debilitating for patients with chronic mold issues) but when it was looked into, my colleague assessed it was actually from vaccine shedding that had contaminated their environment.

•Like the cleaners mentioned earlier, my colleague notices a significant difference in environments that have vs. have not had a significant presence of vaccinated individuals in them.

•Whatever is creating this smell is gradually seeping into the environment (e.g., a colleague through muscle testing recently found the same toxin in seawater foam from the ocean a patient reacted to).

•Not every vaccinated person has an overt shedding smell, but with almost all of them, it can be detected once the air next to them is breathed in.

*Note: I believe this could be explained by the fact only some people received vaccines with positively charged lipid nanoparticles that hence concentrated in the lungs.*

•My colleague believes that whatever is causing this smell behaves a lot like a pheromone. Likewise, Ryan Cole has shared that he believes the pheromonal process is a likely mechanism to account for much of what is being seen with shedding as female menstruation is highly sensitive to pheromones (this reader and this reader also associate shedding with pheromones).

*Note: my colleague (and their mentor) have also found that it is more difficult to treat or evaluated truly vaccinated individuals, as a haze is present around them which makes muscle testing more difficult to perform and their simple presence in the office can interfere with treating other patients who are also there. Initially this forced them to not see vaccinated patients, but in time they found workarounds for this issue. Presently, this colleague and their mentor (who has a good track record in working with complex illness) believes the primary mechanism of toxicity from the shedding is energetic rather than physical in nature (which may for instance explain the experiences of this reader).*

I suspect in the years to come, this smell will become much more clearly worked out. Additionally (assuming it is a physical smell rather than "energetic" smell), I am almost certain it will be possible to train dogs to smell it. For instance, consider (to quote UCLA) what they were able to do with COVID-19:

When the COVID-19 pandemic struck, the diagnostic abilities of dogs were put to the test. Professional trainers claimed high success rates of dogs sniffing out COVID-19 infections, and a few small studies backed them up. In one, specially trained dogs were 97% accurate in sniffing out COVID-19 from sweat samples taken from 335 people. This included finding infection in 31 individuals with no symptoms. When testing moved from isolated biological materials in a lab to actual humans in real-world settings, accuracy dropped a bit.

When it comes to the widespread use of specially trained dogs to diagnose COVID-19, more study is needed. However, researchers and clinicians agree it's a promising avenue. Dogs detected infection up to 48 hours earlier than a PCR test. And while a rapid test requires a swab, chemical reagents and 10 minutes or so to produce results, the dog's response is immediate. There is also interest in harnessing the canine sense of smell to learn more about long COVID.

**Shedding Mechanisms**

*Note: I recently wrote an article titled "*How Do We Navigate Uncertainty In These Perilous Times?*" primarily to provide critical context for this section.*

As I discussed above (and in more detail in the first half of this series), the major issue I've had with this subject is that in theory, mRNA vaccines should not be able to shed, but for some reason they are.

At this point, I've come up with a few ***potentially viabl***e explanation to explain why this is happening. The ones I feel have enough evidence to substantiate them are as follows:

**Variable Sensitivity**

From all the previously received case reports, it has been established that the sensitivity to either the spike protein (or a yet unknown vaccine component) varies by orders of magnitude (discussed further in the first half of this series). While this does not explain how the vaccine is able to "shed" it explains why some people can be relatively unaffected by high concentrations of it (e.g., the asymptomatic shedders) whereas others get very ill from the tiny amount of the shedding agent which exits the body and can be absorbed from the environment.

This in turn is consistent with the hypotheses that the spike protein's toxicity is partly a result of it being an allergen (some people are extraordinarily sensitive to an allergen) and it being an agent which collapses the physiologic zeta potential (as everyone has a differing critical threshold below which impaired zeta potential will trigger microclotting throughout the body).

**Exosome Mediated Shedding**

While not perfect, exosome shedding is the hypothesis that best fits the existing data on shedding. Briefly, this hypothesis argues that the vaccine is concentrating in the lungs (due its previously described affinity for the pulmonary arteries when the vaccine is incorrectly manufactured), which results in some (but not all vaccinated) individuals exhaling a significant amount of spike protein containing exosomes which then affect those in their surrounding. This mode of "shedding transmission" essentially allows for a relatively small difference in total spike protein concentration between the shedder and the individual affected by the shedder.

*Note: Before I learned why the vaccine manufacturing process can cause the vaccine to accumulate in the lungs, I came to suspect something caused the vaccine to concentrate in the arteries that travel from the heart to the lungs because clinicians kept on reporting to me that it seemed to be a primary site of injury in their vaccine injured patients. Likewise, I now suspect the "strongest" shedders were those who received lipid nanoparticles that were manufactured in a way which caused them to concentrate in the lungs.*

Exosomes for reference are small vesicles (which the lipid nanoparticles sought to mimic) that cells continually release and take in, hence forming a critical communication network the entire body relies upon (e.g., mothers have exosomes in their breastmilk which make it through the digestive tract and deliver [micro]RNA to their developing babies which plays a critical epigenetic role in guiding their healthy development). In the same way that mRNA is a relatively new and unexplored technology, the science of exosomes is still in its infancy. Nonetheless, many clinicians are actively using "healthy" exosomes in practice (e.g., those derived from stem cells or amniotic fluid) and having remarkable improvements occur for a variety of degenerative conditions.

During COVID, we noticed that the virus appeared to poison the exosome system and in turn that injecting healthy exosomes into the blood stream often produced remarkable results for those patients (as well as for long COVID and to a lesser extent vaccine injuries). In the case of the vaccine, this makes a lot of sense, as the vaccine works by causing cells to mass produce spike proteins (which get pushed to the cell surface at which point they can bud off into toxic exosomes that traverse the body). In turn, it has been shown this does indeed occur after vaccination (and I suspect, due to the vaccine design, much more frequently than is seen in COVID—which may account for why "vaccine" shedding differs from COVID-19 shedding).

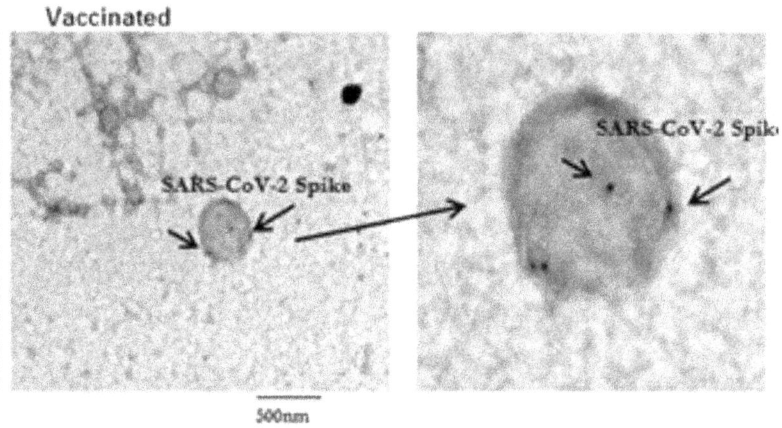


*Note: the negative controls in this experiment did have spike protein on their exosomes.*

Because of all the signaling effects generated by exosomes (very small doses of healthy exosomes can create profound improvements in patients which are hard to believe unless you see it first hand), it in turns seems plausible that inhaling toxic exosomes could have a profound impact on those sensitive to shedding. Furthermore, many of the vaccine injury case histories I've seen indicate the route of exposure had to be respiratory in nature (e.g., the rapid nose bleeds), further supporting this hypothesis. Conversely, I've seen spike protein injured patients have excellent pulmonary and nasal responses to nebulized amniotic exosomes, which again indicates that toxic exosomes could also be active there.

Presently, the following has been shown:

•Spike protein containing exosomes (which circulate in the bloodstream) spike after vaccination (and then decline) and appear to be one of the primary things responsible for triggering the immune response that creates antibodies to the vaccine, as once spike protein coated exosomes are transferred to mice, the mice develop antibodies to the spike protein (along with increasing levels of various inflammatory cytokines).

•A 2023 peer-reviewed study found that unvaccinated children who were around COVID-19 vaccinated parents developed an immune response to the spike protein that was not seen in children with unvaccinated parents. Additionally, they were also able to find spike protein antibodies in surgical masks worn by the physicians. This led the authors to ***hypothesize*** that antibodies being directly transferred through the parent's breath to their children.

I however would argue the results suggest spike coated exosomes (which produce spike antibodies once they arrive in the children) are being transferred. This is because, to the best of my knowledge, it has not otherwise been shown antibodies can be directly transferred to someone else through breath (this would change a lot of the fundamental principles of how herd immunity works in the population) and if the transference were to occur, the concentration in the child would be dramatically lower than the parent (which as best as I can tell was not what the study found).

•Significant amounts of (RNA containing) exosomes can be found in your breath, and those exosomes (which derive from the lungs) vary depending upon on the disease state someone has ("sicker" people have "worse" exosomes). To illustrate, see this 2013 paper, this 2020 paper and this 2021 paper

*Note: since this is a relatively new field of research, each paper is more sophisticated than the preceding one.*

•The spike protein has a high (heparin dependent) affinity for binding to the surface of exosomes. So if was not already there when the exosome initially formed it can also attach to exosomes traveling in the blood stream.

•Long COVID (and more severe acute COVID) is characterized by the presence of more spike protein studded exosomes (see this paper and this paper). Additionally, they also showed exosomes from COVID patients are highly inflammatory (and potentially clot forming) and are taken up by the lung cells. The most detailed study (and imaging) of spike protein containing exosomes can be found in this paper (which also found that spike protein containing exosomes can circulate a year after COVID infection).

*Note: this study also found COVID triggers the production of spike protein coated exosomes, and when lung cells was exposed to those exosomes, an immune response to the spike protein was triggered.*

•An inhaled vaccine was made from lung derived exosomes coated with spike proteins (they were lung derived so the lung cells would be more likely to absorb them). These spike protein exosomes both generated an immune response and were absorbed into the body. Once absorbed, those exosomes then traveled to other tissues and organs in the body which (based on all the reports we've received and the patients we've seen) are known to be affected by shedding.

*Note: the key point from the above studies is that many of the above papers showed (abnormal) exosomes (e.g., spike protein coated ones) activated the immune system and appeared to play a key role in developing an immune response to them.*

Lastly, exosomes may also be absorbed through skin contact (after being sweated out by a shedder) but it's harder to know if this does occur, as the existing data I've seen indicates it's often difficult for (generic) exosomes to penetrate the skin. As there are many cases suggesting skin to skin shedding transmission occurs, that either means something else is at work or spike coated exosomes indeed can penetrate the skin (e.g., because the skin becomes more porous at certain times or because containing spike protein increases the ability of an exosome to penetrate the skin).

In short, I think the theory behind mRNA vaccines (having cells produce exosomes on their surface which are then recognized by the immune system), was a terrible idea since it not only causes the body to attack those potentially essential cells (e.g., a good case can be made this happens to the heart) but also that it poisons the exosome system. This again illustrates why it was a terrible decision to abandon the existing regulatory principles and allow a completely brand new technology with a huge number of unknowns to be given to a large number of people. While the regulators might have wanted to hope those unknowns would all be "fine" as time goes forward, we discover reason after reason they are actually a huge problem.

*Note: The clinical uses of exosomes and their rationale for being used is discussed in much more detail here.*

**The SARS-CoV-2 Virus**

I believe some of the shedding people attribute to the vaccine is in fact due to the virus itself. In turn, there are a few reasons why could happen and it is likely one or more of the following is occurring:

**1.** The SARS-CoV-2 virus is pervasive throughout our environment now and since the shedding symptoms resemble other spike protein injuries, it is likely some of the cases that are being labeled as "shedding" are actually just exposure to the SARS-CoV-2 virus. However, I must note I do not believe this can account for many of the stories I've come across.

**2.** The COVID vaccine transforms the immune response of an injected individual from one that eliminates the infection to one that reduces the symptoms of an existing infection. This in turn may lead to vaccinated individuals becoming chronic "silent" carries of COVID-19 and unawarely shed the virus into their environment. This effect is traditionally observed with vaccines directed at a toxin an infectious agent produces rather than the organism itself (e.g., the pertussis vaccine prevents its toxin from causing whooping cough which can lead to vaccinated individuals becoming chronic carries of pertussis and silently shedding it into their environment—something demonstrated by pertussis outbreaks occurring in vaccinated institutions). In the case of COVID-19 vaccination, it has been discovered that repeated exposure to the (highly allergenic) spike protein triggers the body to begin switching to producing of IgG4 antibodies, antibodies which are reduce the immune response to an allergen—something which is helpful for say pollens you are always exposed to, but not helpful for a harmful agent reproducing within the body.

*Note: I suspect many of the vaccinated individuals predominantly become symptomatic when they are exposed to new variants they do not yet have an IgG4 response to.*

In turn, it appears that repeated vaccination reduces the symptoms from a COVID-19 infection as you no longer have the (often dangerous) allergic response to the spike protein, but it also prolongs the duration of the infection and can turn you into a silent carries of the infection. This again illustrates why it was unwise to deploy a poorly understood technology upon the world and that had a more thorough risk analysis of been performed, people would have realized that it was unwise to perpetually produce the infectious component of SARS-CoV-2 in the body.

*Note: As further proof of this point, Novavax was able to demonstrate that their vaccine (which provides threee injections of the antigen alongside an adjuvant rather than forcing the body to continually produce the spike protein) does not trigger the IgG4 response seen from the mRNA vaccines.*

**3.** Vaccinating someone currently infected with COVID-19 causes the existing infection to spiral out of control, which in turn leads to the infected individual suddenly transmitting large amounts of the pathogen into the environment. Some of the things that have made me suspect this are:

•I personally know of numerous cases (which I logged) where someone got a COVID-19 vaccine, shortly after came down with a severe case of COVID-19 and then died in the hospital.

Likewise, analyses of VAERS reports have found after 1-2 weeks, the most common causes of death reported following vaccination was a

COVID-19 infection.

*Note: I could see this either being due to the immune suppressive effects of the vaccine (e.g., the immune system becoming hyper-primed to respond to the spike protein rather than the existing viral strain, the vaccine being demonstrated to destroy the bone marrow stem cells which produce the immune system's cells or the IgG4 class switch) or due to it provoking a severe inflammatory response (as much of the damage of from a COVID-19 infection is a result of the immunological response to it).*

•I have seen a few reports (e.g., in a survey Steve Kirsch asked me to review) of someone who had a mild (PCR confirmed) lingering COVID infection then get a COVID vaccine and immediately crash (e.g., they needed to be hospitalized). These examples again suggest that the immunosuppressive effects of the vaccine can destroy the immune system's ability to properly respond to an existing infection.

*Note: This was also something that was seen with the HPV vaccine (if you have the HPV strain known to cause cancer at the time you got the vaccine, the HPV trials showed you actually became more likely to get cervical cancer). Since the HPV vaccine and the COVID-19 vaccines are the most immunologically agitating vaccines on the market (e.g., they have a very high rate of causing autoimmune disorders), I suspect they are much more likely to worsen the response to a prexisting infection of the disease they "protect" you against.*

•I know a hermit who I can verify stayed inside his house for the last two years except to see his parents once a week. Throughout the pandemic he never had an issue with COVID, but after his parents were vaccinated, he immediately developed a significant COVID infection. Likewise, I have read numerous reports of people who either came down with COVID or a COVID like illness after being around a vaccinated individual. For example, this was one reader's shedding story:

In December of 2021 we attended a family wedding in another state . We drove there in our RV, not stopping often in restaurants. My husband and I were one of the few at this wedding unvaccinated , which the rest of the family disapproved of , so I was careful in my exposure . We took a home covid test two days before seeing everyone and again on the day we arrived . Negative. At the wedding I was dancing with my nephew , a police officer , who had recently been boosted . He wasn't feeling well - and two days later he tested positive . Three days later , feeling achy and unwell , I tested positive and two days later my husband tested positive. I am sure my nephew was shedding . The only people at the wedding who got sick were relatives or friends of my nephew.

Likewise, another reader shared this story:

My husband and I had the same hair stylist. She said she had just gotten boosted in Feb 2023 (after initial 2 shots). That week, we both got our hair done by her. We both are unvaccinated and had never had Covid. We both came down with Covid that week.

*Note: if you consider the first point, the vaccine could also be causing a chronic COVID infection which causes the vaccinated to continually expel spike protein coated exosomes and those are what actually create the problem for those around them.*

**Bacterial DNA Plasmid Contamination**

It has now been demonstrated that the vaccines are contaminated with DNA plasmids that were not removed during the (improper) manufacturing process.

In turn, I believe it is quite possible those plasmids are in turn integrating into the recipient's genome or their microbiome. Assuming they are in fact integrating into the microbiome, the transfected bacteria will reproduce the spike protein plasmid and can hence transfect other bacteria in the microbiome (which in turn can produce the spike protein). In turn, since we are always spreading our microbiome (including through the air) to those around us, spike transfected bacteria provide a way that the vaccine could allow a replication competent organism to be transmitted to those around us—something which on the surface appears impossible with the mRNA technology (and is hence frequently used to argue against the possibility of shedding).

Presently, the following data points exist to support this hypothesis:

1. It is now known that the most dangerous vaccine lots also had higher amounts of the plasmid contaminants.
2. One system of medicine (based on terrain theory) believes the microbiome transforming into a pathologic state is the root cause of many illnesses. In turn, this system "treats" a variety of diseases by providing plasmids extracted from healthy states of the common organisms found within the body under the theory that unhealthy ones will take up those plasmids, transform into the healthy ones that live with the body and then produce more of the "healthy" plasmids. In essence, this approach seeks to restore health is

exactly the opposite of what the (spike protein plasmid containing) COVID vaccines are doing.

While I do not follow the fairly complex protocols adherents of this school of medicine ask patients to follow, I have found that some of their remedies are extremely helpful for specific diseases that are otherwise quite difficult to treat. With spike protein injuries, we've found one remedy this system believes "treats" the microorganism which causes blood clotting is quite helpful for both vaccine injuries and long-haul COVID. This in turn suggests to us that something about the spike protein pathologically alters the microbiome until it is reversed with a healthy plasmid.

*Note: much more was written about this school of medicine* here.

3. A 2022 study was able to prove that the SARS-CoV-2 virus will infect the gut microbiome, reproduce its components within those bacteria and alter the gut microbiome (due to the bacteria it infected dying). Since bacteriophages typically require specialized proteins to infect bacteria, the fact that SARS-CoV-2 acted as a bacteriophage was a bit of a mystery, which led the study's authors to propose a few ***guesses*** on why it happened, all of which understandably lacked evidence to support them.

4. Sabine Hazan MD, who is a gastroenterologist and a world expert on the microbiome likewise discovered that:

•SARS-CoV-2 could be found in the stools of individuals with a COVID-19 infection.

•That a SARS-CoV-2 infection pathologically altered the gut microbiome.

•That the severity of a COVID-19 infection correlates to the degree of pathologic alteration of the gut microbiome, although it was indeterminate if the alterations in the gut microbiome preceded the infection (and hence predisposed one to a severe infection) or if it was a result of the infection itself.

*Note: this study and this case report suggested that restoring the gut microbiome shortened COVID-19 hospitalization time and significantly improved one's likelihood of survival. Dr. Hazan has also put forth the hypothesis that some of the benefit of ivermectin may be a result of it increasing the beneficial gut bacteria which are harmed by a COVID-19 infection.*

•That mRNA vaccination pathologically altered the gut microbiome (and reduced the same beneficial bacteria observed to be lost in COVID-19 infections, particularly bifidobacteria) both one month after vaccination and at 6-9 months post vaccination.

All of this suggests **but does not prove** that microbiome transfection plays a key role in the shedding phenomenon. One thing that makes me more open to this hypothesis are the numerous cases (e.g., the cleaners discussed in the previous article) I've come across of individuals becoming ill from touching surfaces that were touched by shedders (and hence could contain those spike protein transfected bacteria).

*Note: While it was widely believed to do so throughout the pandemic, SARS-CoV-2 is not transmitted by contaminated surfaces, which means something else is "shedding" onto them. While it's possible it is the spike protein exosomes, it's unclear to me if they could persist in the environment (we always are instructed to store therapeutic exosomes at very low temperatures but in contrast, one study I found suggests serum exosomes can persist at room temperature for a few days) and as mentioned above, it's unclear if they can be absorbed through the skin.*

Additionally, Dr. Hazan's work makes me wonder if the pre-existing microbiome of an individual may influence their susceptibility to shedding.

*Note: I asked Dr. Hazan if she was ever able to assess if vaccination caused the gut microbiome to produce the spike protein. She told me she never had the funding to do the research (as given it's controversial nature, no one wanted to fund it so she had to use up a lot of her savings to self-fund the COVID-19 vaccination studies [that type of research costs a lot]) and she is thus presently trying to raise the funds for the research to determine if the vaccine integrates into the human genome or microbiome (which can be donated to here). While talking to her, she emphasized that the mRNA vaccine damaging the gut microbiome could potentially be creating some of the shedding symptoms being observed since a healthy microbiome both produces essential nutrients and reduces inflammation throughout the body.*

**Pheromones**

As mentioned above, some believe the vaccine shedding pathology is largely mediated through pheromones (hence why some can smell their distinct odor). Ryan Cole endorses this hypothesis, partly because it is known that pheromones can have a significant impact on menstruation. Likewise, a few readers [1,2] have shared that they believe shedders emit a toxic "pheromone." While this possibility is intriguing, I do not believe it can explain everything that has been observed with shedding.

*Note: as far as I know, there is no research on the connection between exosomes and pheromones.*

**Lipid Nanoparticle Breakdown Products**

The shedding is an allergic reaction to the broken down components of the lipid nanoparticles (e.g., PEG) being excreted from patients. Overall, I feel this explanation is unlikely account for much of what has been observed.

**Remaining Questions**

Given how controversial the idea an injection being given to billions of people could actually be actively harming unvaccinated people is, we've put a lot of thought into if we wanted to broach this topic. For this reason, we've spent a long time researching the topic and tried to stick to claims we could provide the evidence to substantiate.

At this point, I feel we have been able to answer many of the questions numerous people have asked us to explore. Nonetheless, there are a few topics that have not yet been covered I know many of you still want some guidance on. The dilemma we face is that most of those answers rely more speculative evidence and our fear is that if they are associate with these points, they will be focused on and hence used to dismiss the rest of the critically important points raised throughout this article.

For example, many people want to know how to protect themselves from shedding. In my eyes, the best answer to this question is the same message everyone in this movement has been giving for the last year: "stop boosting people." However, since we are still not at that point (however we are close as most of the public appears to have realized the boosters are either unsafe or ineffective), I am not sure if that constitutes useful advice. Likewise, I think making people conscious of how shedding may be harming them is helpful since it provides guidance on how to significantly reduce that harm by avoiding shedding exposures, but at the same time it's not really helpful because no one wants to be stuck being isolated from society (which many readers here have shared is the situation they've now found themselves in).

*Note: I am hopeful the shedding issue, provided it's presented in a reasonable and measured manner, may finally be the thing that tips the scales against continuing the COVID-19 booster campaign as the incentives to keep them on the market is rapidly dwindling (since almost no one is buying them).*

In the final part of this article, I will attempt to answer the more challenging questions that still lie on much shakier ground. Specifically:

- What can be done to mitigate the effects of shedding that cannot be avoided?
- What do we currently know about shedding and sexual relationships?

•What do we currently know about shedding and cancer?

•What do we currently know about shedding and blood transfusions from vaccinated individuals?

•What are the more controversial mechanisms for shedding that are currently being considered?

The entirety of the article can be found online @ https://www.midwesterndoctor.com/p/unraveling-the-mystery-of-mrna-vaccine?utm_source=publication-search
Including new and expanded studies in this area.

# A Few Words from the Author

I have endeavored to provide reliable resources, history and facts that I hope make sense, are compiled well and provide irrefutable evidence that vaccines never were and still are not the answer to better health or a better future.

While I have personally had my doubts about vaccines for decades, I still had to reframe my ideas about how disease works and eliminate my fears that led me to compromise in this area of health.

As one who has been partially vaccinated myself (as most of the world has, sadly) and watched firsthand the results of seeing my children vaxxed/unvaxxed, I can personally vouch for the claims I make about my own observations and others that I have witnessed.

My journey of understanding disease processes and the science behind what is currently taking place is constantly evolving and I am committed to keeping an open mind and simply doing my best to understand and accept truth in an unbiased way (we all have our bias). I do believe that history, true history, is the best teacher we have to properly interpret the present.

At the end, I want what (I hope) we all want: to secure a better and eternally beautiful future for ourselves and our children. We all have different ideas about how to get there. I believe firmly we will never arrive unless we can take hold of truth in each generation and have the humility to concede our own opinions and viewpoints for what has proven to be a greater reality.

Truly, if we cut through to the root of the issue, our quest for what is GOOD in every area is a pursuit of finding God, our creator, and ourselves in the very truest sense, which is the only thing that can allow us to succeed on the path of life.

I wish you every blessing and success in this endeavor. Together.

Rachel Banura

www.ingramcontent.com/pod-product-compliance
Lightning Source LLC
Chambersburg PA
CBHW052119270326
41930CB00012B/2682
*9798999183811*